gas
laser
technology

gas
laser
technology

DOUGLAS C. SINCLAIR
W. EARL BELL

HOLT, RINEHART AND WINSTON, INC.
New York   Chicago   San Francisco   Atlanta
Dallas   Montreal   Toronto   London   Sydney

Library of Congress Catalog Card Number: 69-13796
SBN: 03-075385-6

Printed in the United States of America

01234   22   98765432

To our families, not only
for their help during the preparation of this book,
but also for their emphatic understanding of
lasers that don't lase.

PREFACE

During the past few years, a new field of scientific endeavor has begun, a field that we call "gas-laser technology." It has been an exciting field to work in, both because of the fascinating characteristics of gas lasers themselves, and because of the challenges posed by the demands of gas-laser technology requiring simultaneous advances in several existing disciplines.

Although, on a historical scale, the field is undoubtedly in its infancy, there now exists a substantial body of knowledge that those who are continuing work in the field should be familiar with. Our book is an attempt to present an epitome of this work.

The book is generally meant for people who want to know about and work with gas lasers. We have tried to describe the material at a level that we consider most appropriate for communication. The discussion should certainly be comprehensible to doctoral students embarking on thesis research in engineering or physics, and much of it can be understood by advanced undergraduates.

We have, in our discussion, tried to paraphrase, rather than summarize, the literature. There are two reasons for this: The first is that a strict summary of the literature would seem of little more value than a bibliography; the second is that, in the course of working in a field for several years, one develops personal viewpoints concerning the ways that one feels a subject "ought" to be treated. We hope that ours match those of the reader.

Because of our approach, the reference section at the end of each chapter should be of particular value. We have chosen to list only a few references, and to include comments on what they contain. This has prevented us from referencing as many papers as we would have liked to; there are, however, extensive bibliographies in the papers which we do reference in this book, and the reader who wants to pursue individual subjects in greater detail than given in this book will find these bibliographies helpful.

The relative paucity of references in this book should not be interpreted as a lack of acknowledgment of the work of others. One of the delightful aspects of working in the field of gas-laser technology has been the free exchange of ideas among scientists throughout the world. One of us (D. C. S.) would like to pay special tribute to his former colleagues at the Institute of Optics, University of Rochester, and both of us would like to pay tribute to our colleagues at Spectra-Physics, with whom we have had daily contact. In addition to these people, however, are hundreds of others with whom we have had discussions during the past few years. It is the summation of all this interaction that has taught us what we know about gas-laser technology. We hope that in this book we are successful in communicating this knowledge to others.

Palo Alto, California   DOUGLAS C. SINCLAIR
                                                                          W. EARL BELL

CONTENTS

SYMBOLS

The following is a summary of symbols used in the text. The numbers following the symbol descriptions are page references.

A	field amplitude, 49	G_0'	unsaturated gain including collisions, 42
A_n	temporal eigenfunction, 38	g_l	gain per unit length (gain coefficient), 5
a	mirror loss, 114		
$-a, a$	mirror width, 64	g_{l0}	unsaturated gain coefficient at line center in the absence of line broadening, 30
a, b	energy-level expansion coefficients, 16		
b	confocal radius of curvature, 71		
b'	beam parameter, 78	g_t	gain per unit time (temporal gain coefficient), 6
c	$2\pi \times$ Fresnel number, 72		
c	velocity of light, 6	g_{t0}	unsaturated temporal gain coefficient at line center in the absence of line broadening, 39
d	diameter, 8		
E	electric intensity, 16		
E_a, E_b	energy of state a or b, 16	H	Hamiltonian, 16
		H_m, H_n	Hermite polynomials, 73
E_n	amplitude of temporal eigenfunction, 38	$\mathbf{H}$	Hamiltonian matrix, 19
E_0	amplitude of electric intensity, 22	$\hbar$	Planck's constant, 16
		$\mathscr{I}_m$	spatial Fourier component of inversion density, 55
F, F'	lateral focal points, 78		
f	focal length, 89		
$f^{\#}$	f number, 94	$\mathscr{I}_0$	inversion density, 24
G	gain, 6	i	$\sqrt{-1}$, 20

k	Boltzmann's constant, 29	u_m, v_n	scalar optical field, 64
k, K	wave number $2\pi/\lambda$, 41	V_{int}	interaction potential, 16
L	length, 5	v	velocity, 29
$L_p{}^l$	Laguerre polynomial, 96	W	intensity (power per unit area), 5
L_T	threshold length, 43	W_s	saturation parameter, 45
M	atomic mass, 29	W_{s0}	saturation parameter, 25
m, n	transverse mode numbers, 64	w_0	spot size at beam waist, 84
N	Fresnel number, 65	w_s	spot size, 74
N	number of atoms per unit volume, 19	X	excitation parameter, 47
n	integer, 9	x, y	distance, 64
n	refractive index, 24	Z, Z_r, Z_i	plasma dispersion function, 31
n_a, n_b	average number of atoms per unit volume in state a or b, 23	z	distance, 37
n_1, n_2	refractive indices, 91	α_m	Lamb coefficient, 50
P	electric polarization, 25	α_t	loss per unit time (temporal loss coefficient), 37
P	probability, 16		
P_{out}	output power, 120	β_m	Lamb coefficient, 50
p	dipole moment, 16	$\boldsymbol{\Gamma}$	decay matrix, 20
Q	quality factor, 37	γ_a, γ_b	decay rates of state a or b, 17
q	longitudinal mode number, 73	γ	average decay rate, 18
R	radius of curvature of wavefront or mirror, 75, 82	γ_s	saturated decay rate, 25
R	rate constant, 23	γ'	average decay rate including collision effects, 28
r	distance, 64		
r	reflectance, 37	γ'_s	collision-broadened saturated decay rate, 28
S_{0n}, R_{0n}	wave functions in prolate spheroidal coordinates, 72	$\gamma, \gamma_m, \gamma_n$	mode eigenvalue, 63
S_1	mirror surface area, 64	Δ	angular difference frequency between two cavity resonances, 49
T	temperature, 29		
t	integration variable, 30	$\Delta\omega_D$	Doppler width of spectral line, 29
t	mirror transmission, 114	ϵ_0	permittivity of free space, 25
t	time, 16	η	broadening parameter, 30
U_n	spatial eigenfunction, 37		

η_{mn}	Lamb coefficient, 52	ρ_m	Lamb coefficient, 52
ϑ	divergence angle, 8	$\boldsymbol{\rho}$	density matrix, 19
ϑ	obliquity angle, 64	σ	propagation-circle designator, 78
ϑ	phase angle, 41		
ϑ_{mn}	Lamb coefficient, 52	σ_m	Lamb coefficient, 52
Λ_a, Λ_b	excitation rates to state a or b, 23	τ_{mn}	Lamb coefficient, 52
		Φ	phase angle, 75
λ	wavelength, 8	φ	phase angle, 38
$\boldsymbol{\lambda}$	excitation matrix, 21	χ', χ''	real and imaginary parts of complex susceptibility, 24
λ_a, λ_b	excitation matrix elements, 21		
μ	dipole matrix element, 17	ψ	relative phase angle, 52
		ψ	wave function, 16
$\bar{\mu}$	ensemble-averaged dipole matrix element, 19	Ω	angular frequency of cavity resonance, 36
ξ	normalized frequency, 30	ω	angular frequency, 9
ξ_{mn}	Lamb coefficient, 52	ω_0	angular frequency of transition between states a and b, 18
π	propagation-circle designator, 78		
ρ	distance, 75	ω'	Doppler-shifted angular frequency, 29
ρ_{ab}	element of density matrix, 19, 22	ω_{12}	$(\omega_1 + \omega_2)/2$, 55

1 INTRODUCTION

A gas laser is a light source. In its most common form, it consists of (1) a gas discharge that can amplify light and (2) a pair of high-reflectance mirrors. A typical gas laser is illustrated schematically in Figure 1-1.

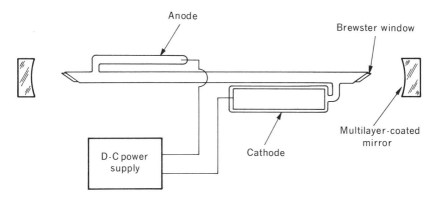

FIG. 1-1. Typical gas-laser configuration.

The laser mirrors are usually spherical and are coated with multilayer dielectric films having a reflectance on the order of 99 percent. The tube containing the gas discharge is known as a "plasma tube." The ends of the plasma tube are terminated by windows, called "Brewster windows," which are placed on the tube so that the angle between the normal to the windows and the axis of the plasma tube is equal to Brewster's angle.[1] At this angle,

---

[1] Brewster's angle is equal to the arctangent of the refractive index of the window and is typically about 56°.

1

light which is linearly polarized in the plane of incidence will pass through the windows with no loss due to Fresnel reflection. It is therefore possible to construct a plasma tube, separate from the laser mirrors, that introduces very little optical loss; this represents a great convenience, because it permits the experimenter to interchange the mirrors on a laser easily. Lasers which are not designed for experimental use are often constructed with the mirrors fastened directly to the plasma tube.

If the amplification of light by the gas discharge exceeds the loss at the mirrors, the system will be regenerative and will function as a "light oscillator."[2]

The initial build-up of the laser oscillation is triggered by the spontaneous emission of light having the proper frequency, direction, and polarization. The requisite frequency is defined by two conditions: (1) the frequency must be within the "linewidth" of a radiative transition which exhibits amplification, and (2) the frequency must be such that the "optical cavity" defined by the laser mirrors is resonant. The direction is defined by the optical axis of the mirror system, and the polarization is defined by the Brewster windows: the optical loss will be least for light incident on the Brewster windows which is linearly polarized in the plane of incidence; this polarization will dominate over all other polarizations.

Light which is spontaneously emitted as described above will stimulate the emission of additional light. The intensity[3] of the oscillation in the laser will then build up to the point where the power contributed to the oscillator by the gas discharge is equal to the power lost by the mirrors. In a steady-state oscillation, the amplification must saturate so that the gain is equal to the loss. To be strictly correct, one should note that in a steady-state oscillation the gain will be slightly less than the loss, because there will always be some spontaneous emission occurring; however, the ratio of the spontaneous emission power to the stimulated emission power is extremely small, and spontaneous emission can usually be neglected once the laser is oscillating. The presence of spontaneous emission gives rise to "noise" on the laser beam.

The output beam from the laser is obtained by making one of the mirrors partially transmitting. The maximum output power will be obtained when all

---

[2] It was suggested in the early 1960s that the name "laser," which is an acronym for "*l*ight *a*mplification by *s*timulated *e*mission of *r*adiation," should be changed to "loser," since most lasers were used as oscillators. It was decided, however, that it would be difficult to obtain funding for research on "losers," and the suggestion was dropped.

[3] The term "intensity" will be used in this book to mean the power per unit area in an electromagnetic field. The magnitude of the square root of the intensity will be called the "amplitude" of the field.

the light not reflected by the laser mirrors is transmitted through them; absorption and scattering losses in the mirrors are detrimental to obtaining a high output power.

The mirrors must be aligned so that the optical axis defined by them (which is determined by the line connecting their centers of curvature) passes through the plasma tube; in an ideal situation, the optical axis would coincide with the plasma-tube axis. The alignment tolerance of the mirrors depends on their radius of curvature: the maximum alignment tolerance will be obtained when the radius of curvature of the mirrors is slightly less than their separation; the minimum alignment tolerance will be obtained when the mirrors are either flat or have a radius of curvature equal to one-half their separation. If the radius of curvature of the mirrors is less than one-half their separation, the diffraction loss of light reflected back and forth between them will be excessive, and the laser usually will not oscillate.

The excitation of the gas is usually accomplished by either a direct-current or a radio-frequency discharge. There are many factors that influence the choice of a discharge scheme; but to a first approximation, the characteristics of the laser do not depend on the method used to excite the discharge.

The *sine qua non* of a laser is a transition which amplifies, rather than absorbs, light. Such transitions are not easily found; in a gas which is in thermal equilibrium, lower-lying energy levels will be more heavily populated than higher-lying energy levels, and light incident on such a gas will be absorbed rather than amplified. Fortunately, the atoms in many gas discharges are not in thermal equilibrium, and several hundred amplifying transitions have been discovered.

In this chapter, we shall consider the general nature of the emission and absorption of light by gas discharges, and we shall describe the most basic characteristics of helium-neon, argon-ion, and carbon dioxide lasers. Our purpose in this chapter is mainly to acquaint the reader with the salient aspects of gas-laser technology. In succeeding chapters, the specific aspects of the subject will be considered in greater detail.

1–1 EMISSION AND ABSORPTION OF LIGHT BY GAS DISCHARGES

There are a wide variety of electronic processes which occur in gas discharges. For our present purposes, it is sufficient to consider only the most elementary processes occurring in a simple direct-current discharge.

In a direct-current gas discharge, electrons are emitted by the cathode. Near the cathode of a direct-current discharge is a region in which there is a moderately high potential gradient: this region of the discharge is called the "cathode-fall" region. Near the anode of a direct-current discharge, gas atoms are ionized and electrons pass from the discharge into the anode. This is also a region of moderately high potential gradient; it is called the "anode-fall" region of the discharge.

The cathode-fall and anode-fall regions of the discharge occur quite close to the cathode and anode, respectively, of the discharge tube. Between these two regions is an extended region called the "positive column." The characteristics of the discharge are essentially constant in this region. The potential gradient is constant, so that there are equal numbers of electrons and ions per unit volume. In the positive column, ions are typically created by collisions of neutral atoms with electrons or ions. They then drift toward the walls of the discharge tube, where they recombine with electrons to form neutral atoms. The positive-column region of a gas discharge is the region in which laser action is usually obtained.

There are a large number of processes which can cause the population of excited states of atoms in the positive column of a gas discharge. The most common excitation process involves an inelastic collision between a moving electron and a ground-state atom. If an electron has a kinetic energy that is equal to or greater than the potential energy of an excited state of a gas atom, an inelastic collision can occur between the electron and an atom; the atom is left in an excited state, and the electron loses an amount of kinetic energy equal to the potential energy of the atom's excited state. This is called a "collision of the first kind," and it is one of the most important processes by which atoms in a gas discharge are excited.

The reverse of the above process can also occur: an excited atom can collide with a slow electron and lose its potential energy to the electron, which emerges from the collision with an additional kinetic energy equal to the excitation potential of the atomic excited state. This is a collision of the second kind.

The term "collision of the second kind" is also applied to a collision in which an excited atom collides with an atom in its ground state, thereby transferring its potential energy to the potential energy of the other atom. This type of process is frequently important in gas lasers.

Another excitation process which occurs in gas discharges is excitation by resonance trapping. In this process, a quantum of light emitted by one atom is absorbed by a different atom, so that the new atom is left in an excited state.

There are three different types of interaction phenomena between an atom and a radiation field. These are spontaneous emission, stimulated emission, and absorption. Spontaneous emission is the radiation process that accounts for the light emitted by an ordinary light source. When an atom is excited to some energy level above its ground state, it can, in general, spontaneously emit a quantum of radiation having an energy equal to the excitation potential of the excited state and thereby return to its ground state.[4] On the other hand, if the excited atom is located in a radiation field having a frequency equal to the excitation potential of the atom (divided by Planck's constant), it can emit a quantum of radiation by stimulated emission. The difference between spontaneous emission and stimulated emission is that spontaneous emission can occur in any direction, and its frequency need only be approximately equal to the excitation potential of the excited state (divided by Planck's constant); whereas stimulated emission must occur in the same direction, with the same polarization, and at the exact frequency of the incident radiation field. To be precise, one should say that the stimulated quantum is in the same "radiation mode" as the quantum that stimulated it.

Absorption is an interaction process which is analogous to stimulated emission. If a radiation field (of the proper frequency) is incident on an atom in its ground state, it can "stimulate" the atom to absorb a quantum of energy from the field. The atom will then be left in an excited state.

In order to maintain thermodynamic equilibrium between matter and a radiation field, the a priori probability of stimulated emission must be exactly equal to the a priori probability of absorption. In most ordinary light sources, the only one of these two processes which is observed experimentally is absorption. The reason for this is that, in most ordinary light sources, the number of atoms in low-energy levels is far greater than the number in high-energy levels. There are thus more atoms available for absorption than there are for stimulated emission, and absorption is observed as the dominant process.

In a laser, the situation is quite different: the number of atoms in some high-energy level is greater than the number in some lower energy level. Such a situation is called a "population inversion."

The existence of a population inversion between two energy levels connected by a radiative transition gives rise to the phenomenon of optical gain. Optical gain is described by parameters analogous to those used to describe optical absorption. If a beam of light having intensity W_1 passes through a length L of an amplifying gas having a gain per unit length[5] g_l, the intensity W_2 of the beam emerging from the gas will be

$$W_2 = W_1 e^{g_l L} \qquad (1\text{-}1)$$

---

[4] Whether or not the transition can actually take place depends on spectroscopic "selection rules," which will not be considered here. Also, the transition need not be directly to the ground state, but merely to a lower energy level.

[5] The gain per unit length is often called the "gain coefficient."

The total gain of a length L of the gas can be written as

$$G = 4.34 g_l L \qquad (1\text{-}2)$$

where G is expressed in decibels.

In describing gas-laser oscillations, it is often convenient to describe amplification in terms of a gain per unit time rather than a gain per unit length. Since light travels with a velocity c, the gain per unit time g_t is related to the gain per unit length g_l by

$$g_t = c g_l \qquad (1\text{-}3)$$

Combining Eqs. (1-2) and (1-3), we see that the total gain (in decibels) experienced by a light wave in passing through an amplifying material of length L is

$$G = 4.34 g_t \frac{L}{c} \qquad (1\text{-}4)$$

The usefulness of the concept of a gain per unit time occurs primarily when one wishes to describe the amplification of standing-wave fields, such as those occurring in gas lasers. This concept will be described further in Chapter 3.

1–2 GAS-LASER SPECTROSCOPY

Since gas lasers are essentially spectroscopic light sources, and since atomic spectroscopy is a well-understood subject, one might expect that the spectroscopic aspects of gas-laser physics would be amenable to detailed theoretical analysis. In reality, such is not generally the case.

The subject of gas-laser spectroscopy can be subdivided into three fairly distinct areas. The first of these concerns the identification of known gas-laser transitions and the assignment of these transitions to the energy levels of atomic systems. This part of gas-laser spectroscopy is comparatively simple, although several laser transitions have been observed (particularly in ion lasers and infrared molecular lasers) which have not yet been assigned to known energy levels.

The second area of gas-laser spectroscopy concerns the prediction of suitable transitions for laser action, and the general characteristics of lasers employing such transitions. In this area, theoretical analysis has been notably unsuccessful. The reason for this is that such analyses must include the various excitation processes which occur in gas discharges, as well as the optical properties of the different atomic energy levels involved. The complexity of the problem is great; and with very few exceptions, all theoretical analyses have failed.

The third area of gas-laser spectroscopy concerns the prediction of the performance of gas lasers when one knows the excitation rates and optical characteristics of a laser transition from experimental data. In this area, considerable progress has been made during the past few years. The principal emphasis on gas-laser spectroscopy in this book will be devoted to a discussion of this third area; only cursory attention will be paid to the first two areas.

1-3 HELIUM-NEON LASERS

The first gas laser to be demonstrated experimentally was the helium-neon laser, which was announced by Javan, Bennett, and Herriott in 1961. The helium-neon laser is still the most widely used gas laser; it is moderately easy to construct and is fairly reliable. It has been more thoroughly studied than any other gas laser, and at the time of this writing its operation is better understood than that of any other gas laser.

The energy levels pertinent to the helium-neon laser are shown in Figure 1-2. The laser transitions occur between various excited states in the neutral spectrum of neon. Of the many wavelengths at which oscillation has been observed, three are of principal importance: 6328 Å, 1.15 μ, and 3.39 μ.

The first transition on which laser oscillation was experimentally observed was the $2s_2 \rightarrow 2p_4$ transition at 1.15 μ. The $2s_2$ state in a pure neon discharge is heavily populated by a combination of collisions of the first kind and resonance trapping. In a helium-neon mixture, the population of the $2s_2$ state is enhanced by collisions of the second kind between helium (metastable) $^3S_1$ atoms and ground-state neon atoms. The $3s_2$ state in neutral neon is also populated by collisions of the second kind between helium (metastable) $^1S_1$ atoms and ground-state neon atoms. It is, in fact, also possible to obtain a population inversion on the $3s_2 \rightarrow 2p_4$ transition at 6328 Å, and on $3s_2 \rightarrow 3p_4$ transition at 3.39 μ.

The output from a helium-neon visible laser is a low-divergence red beam of light. One of the most striking characteristics of this beam is the granular appearance of the light scattered from a diffuse surface (such as a white card placed in the beam). The granular appearance is caused by the spatial coherence of the laser beam.

When spatially coherent light is scattered from a diffuse surface, it forms a random interference pattern throughout space. In front of the surface, the interference pattern is real, and it can be observed on a screen placed near the diffuse surface. Behind the surface, the interference pattern is virtual.

When looking at the red spot formed by a helium-neon laser beam falling on a diffuse surface, one normally focuses slightly behind the surface because

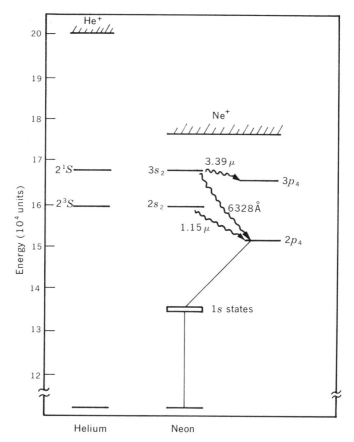

FIG. 1-2.   Energy-level diagram for the helium-neon laser.

of chromatic aberration in the eye. What is seen, therefore, is the virtual random interference pattern caused by the scattered light. With a blue laser, the effect is reversed; chromatic aberration in the eyes causes one to focus slightly in front of the scattering surface. (The plane on which the eyes are focused can be determined by moving one's head from side to side and noting the apparent motion of the granularity due to the effect of parallax.)

Another prominent feature of the laser beam is its low divergence. The divergence of a laser beam is limited solely by diffraction. If the beam emerging from the laser has a diameter d, its angular divergence is given roughly by

$$\vartheta \approx \frac{\lambda}{d} \tag{1-5}$$

where λ is the wavelength of the laser transition.

The above remark needs to be qualified somewhat: we assume that the wavefront of the beam emerging from the laser is plane and that the beam has a gaussian intensity distribution as shown in Figure 1-3a.

In a practical helium-neon laser, the above conditions are usually satisfied. Occasionally, however, a complicated radiation pattern, such as that shown in Figure 1-3b, is obtained. This pattern represents a so-called "high-order transverse mode." Such a pattern is analogous to a microwave-antenna

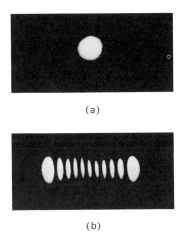

(a)

(b)

FIG. 1-3.   (a) TEM$_{00}$ transverse mode; (b) TEM$_{10,0}$ transverse mode.

pattern, or a mode of a microwave cavity; it is, in fact, a mode of the optical cavity formed by the laser mirrors. When such a pattern is obtained, the value of d to be used in relation (1-5) is approximately (but not exactly) equal to the diameter of one of the lobes of the pattern. A simple gaussian intensity distribution is called a "TEM$_{00}$ transverse mode"; transverse modes are designated by the notation TEM$_{mn}$, where m and n are integers describing the amplitude variations across the beam. For example, the mode shown in Figure 1-3b is a TEM$_{10,0}$ transverse mode.

If the laser beam is detected by a photodetector, the photocurrent will often contain signals having frequencies[6]

$$\omega = n\pi \frac{c}{L} \qquad (1\text{-}6)$$

where n is an integer, c is the velocity of light, and L is the separation between

[6] In this book, frequencies will be designated as angular frequencies; however, numerical values will always be cited as linear frequencies.

the laser mirrors. These signals are caused by the fact that light from the laser is not monochromatic but contains several discrete frequencies separated by the difference frequency given by Eq. (1-6). When the laser beam is detected, these different frequencies "beat" with one another to produce radio-frequency signals in the output photocurrent. By measuring the maximum frequency of the beat signals, the number of different optical frequencies in the laser beam can be deduced. The different optical frequencies that give rise to beats described above are called different "longitudinal modes" of the laser. The amplification bandwidth of a helium-neon visible laser is on the order of 1.5 GHz; this sets an upper limit on the number of longitudinal modes for a fixed-length laser.

The helium-neon laser is inherently a low-power device; typical output powers of helium-neon visible lasers run from about 1 to 100 mW, and somewhat less power is obtained on the infrared transitions.

1-4 ION LASERS

Laser oscillation has been obtained in the ion spectrum of several elements. More than 200 ion-laser transitions have been observed in pulsed-discharge tubes, and several tens of these have been observed to oscillate "cw" (that is, continuously). The most important ion laser currently is the argon laser, which will be described in this section.

The pertinent energy levels of argon are shown in Figure 1-4. Population inversions are obtained between several energy levels in the Ar(II) spectrum. The most important laser transitions are the $4p\,^2D_{5/2}^{\,0} \to 4s\,^2P_{3/2}$ transition at 4880 Å and the $4p\,^4D_{5/2}^{\,0} \to 4s\,^2P_{3/2}$ transition at 5145 Å.

The excitation mechanism of the argon-ion laser is not yet completely understood. It is generally believed that the primary excitation process involves collisions of the first kind and that multiple-collision effects are important.

The population inversion obtained on the 4880-Å transition is large (for a visible transition): gain coefficients in excess of 20 dB/m have been measured in pulsed lasers, and gain coefficients of 3 dB/m are typical for cw lasers.

The cw output power on the 4880-Å and the 5145-Å transitions typically ranges from a fraction of a watt to several watts, and peak output powers of several tens of watts are typically obtained from pulsed lasers.

The essential characteristics of the output beam from an argon-ion laser are similar to those of the output beam from a helium-neon laser. The principal differences between the two output beams are that an argon-ion laser beam has a shorter wavelength, (typically) higher power, and a broader overall linewidth than does a helium-neon laser beam.

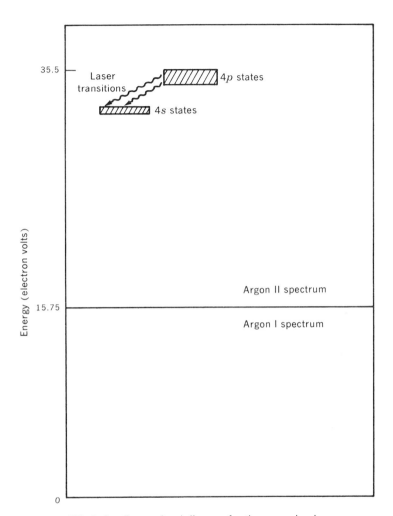

FIG. 1-4.   Energy-level diagram for the argon-ion laser.

1-5 CARBON DIOXIDE LASERS

The highest-power cw gas laser currently available is the carbon dioxide laser, which oscillates on several transitions in the infrared, the principal one having a wavelength of approximately 10.6 μ. Typical output powers of carbon dioxide lasers range from several watts to a few kilowatts and are determined primarily by the amount of electrical power available and the tolerable size of the laser.

An outstanding feature of the carbon dioxide laser is its high efficiency: it is possible to convert electrical power to laser output power with an efficiency of greater than 10 percent.

The pertinent energy levels of carbon dioxide are shown in Figure 1-5. The details of the excitation mechanism are not completely understood at this

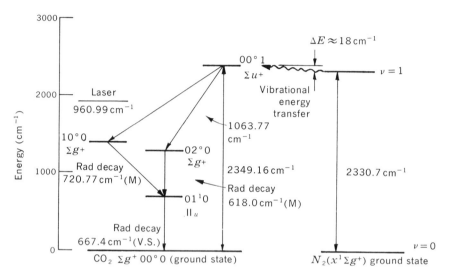

FIG. 1-5.   Energy-level diagram for the CO_2 laser. [*From C. K. N. Patel, Phys. Rev. Letters*, **13**:617 (1964).]

time; apparently a major excitation process involves collisions of the first kind which directly populate the upper laser state. To obtain high output powers from carbon dioxide lasers, it is necessary to add other gases to the discharge. The two most common "additives" are nitrogen and helium. The enhancement obtained from the nitrogen is believed to be caused by population of the upper laser state by collisions of the second kind between metastable nitrogen molecules and ground-state carbon dioxide molecules. The effect of helium on the carbon dioxide laser is apparently to increase the decay rate of the lower laser state by collisional transfer of energy.

The characteristics of the output beam from a carbon dioxide laser are, in principle, similar to those of other gas lasers, but the high power of a carbon dioxide laser often gives rise to effects that are qualitatively different from those obtained with other gas lasers. For example, the usual result obtained when a carbon dioxide laser beam is scattered from a white card is that the card bursts into flame; the details of coherent scattering are of little interest in this case.

REFERENCES

1. W. R. Bennett, Jr., *Appl. Optics Suppl. on Optical Masers*, **1962**: 24; W. R. Bennett, Jr., *Appl. Optics Suppl. on Chem. Lasers*, **1965**: 3; A. L. Bloom, *Appl. Optics*, **5**: 1500 (1966).

These three papers are review articles which summarize progress in the general field of gas lasers. They are well written, and should be read by everyone interested in gas lasers.

2. W. B. Bridges and A. N. Chester, *IEEE J. Quantum Electronics*, **QE-1**: 66 (1965); E. I. Gordon, E. F. Labuda, R. C. Miller, and C. E. Webb, in P. L. Kelley (ed.), "Physics of Quantum Electronics," p. 664, McGraw-Hill Book Company, New York, 1966; E. F. Labuda, E. I. Gordon, and R. C. Miller, *IEEE J. Quantum Electronics*, **QE-1**: 273 (1965).

The papers by Gordon et al. discuss excitation mechanisms and operating characteristics of ion lasers. The article by Bridges and Chester describes the various ionic transitions on which laser action has been obtained.

3. C. K. N. Patel, *J. chim. Phys.*, **1967**: 82.

This is a recent summary of the state of CO_2 laser development. It is not comprehensive; much of the background work is described in the references cited at the end of the paper.

4. E. F. Labuda and E. I. Gordon, *J. Appl. Phys.*, **35**: 1647 (1964); A. D. White and E. I. Gordon, *Appl. Phys. Letters*, **3**: 197 (1963); E. I. Gordon and A. D. White, *Appl. Phys. Letters*, **3**: 199 (1963).

These three papers describe the detailed excitation mechanisms and scaling laws for the helium-neon visible laser, a subject which is not described in this book. They are important papers, although they have apparently been overlooked by many workers. Among other things, they show that the widespread belief that the output power of helium-neon lasers is limited by neon metastable states is erroneous.

2 INTERACTION OF RADIATION AND MATTER

2–1 METHOD OF APPROACH

There are three theoretical approaches commonly used to describe the interaction of radiation and matter: the "thermodynamic" theory, the "semiclassical" theory, and the "quantum" theory.

The simplest of these is the thermodynamic theory, the basic tenets of
which were first stated by Einstein in 1917. For matter to exist in thermal
equilibrium with a radiation field, three types of interaction processes must
occur: (1) matter may absorb radiation; (2) it may emit radiation spontaneously; or (3) it may be forced to give off radiation by stimulated emission.
The detailed balancing of these processes leads to a set of "rate equations"
which govern the interaction between radiation and matter in the thermodynamic theory. The fundamental defect in the theory is that it does not account
for coherence effects in the radiation field. Coherence effects are often important in the emission of radiation by gas lasers, however, and an adequate
theory must describe them.

The semiclassical theory of radiation does account for coherence effects.
The semiclassical theory considers radiation as a classical electromagnetic
field, and matter as a quantum-mechanical system. When radiation is incident
on a material, it induces a dipole moment in the material. In the semiclassical
theory of radiation, the expectation value of the quantum-mechanical dipole
moment is interpreted as a classical polarization. This polarization is then
regarded as a "source" which drives the electromagnetic field. Thus, in the
semiclassical theory, Maxwell's equations govern the field, and Schroedinger's
equation governs the material system.

In the quantum theory of radiation, both the field and the material system
are regarded as quantum systems. Their interaction is governed by the laws

of quantum electrodynamics. The quantum theory and the semiclassical theory are fundamentally different in outlook, although the laser phenomena that they predict are almost always the same.

In this book, the semiclassical theory is adopted for pragmatic reasons: it gives an adequate description of the operation of gas lasers by using concepts which are easy to visualize. In fact, much of our discussion is devoted to the thermodynamic theory. However, instead of describing the thermodynamic theory in terms of the formalism introduced by Einstein, it will be considered here as the "rate-equation approximation" to the semiclassical theory. By approaching the thermodynamic theory in this manner, one can clearly define the limits of its validity.

In this chapter, the formalism and basic equations used in the semiclassical theory of radiation will be developed. This formalism (in the rate-equation approximation) will then be used to determine the gain coefficient[1] and the refractive index of a gas discharge.

One of the main objectives of our analysis will be to determine the manner in which the gain coefficient saturates. Saturation effects are of fundamental importance in gas lasers. If the amplification of radiation in the gas were to exceed the loss in the optical cavity, the intensity of a laser oscillation would increase until it has an infinite magnitude. Clearly this cannot happen in an actual laser; the gain must saturate so that at some finite oscillation intensity the gain equals the loss. A laser (at least when it is used as an oscillator) is thus inherently a nonlinear device.

In order to determine the gain coefficient for a gas, one must choose a model for a gas atom. Any real gas atom has, of course, many energy levels which in a gas discharge are continually being excited and deexcited by an enormous variety of processes. To attempt to consider all the levels or all the excitation processes would result in hopeless complication; therefore, an approximate model will be considered. In particular, a gas comprising atoms which have only two *excited* energy levels of interest will be examined here. These energy levels are excited by some process (or processes) which can be characterized by an "excitation rate." They decay by stimulated emission, by spontaneous emission, or by nonradiative (collisional) processes. The exact nature of these processes is of no interest in the present discussion; it need only be assumed that they can be characterized by a "collisional decay rate."

---

[1] Since this book is about lasers, it seems appropriate to discuss the "gain coefficient" rather than the "absorption coefficient." The two coefficients are related by one being the negative of the other.

Clearly, the gain coefficient of a gas cannot be determined from first principles by using the above model. However, if the values for the various excitation and decay rates which enter into this discussion are known, one may hope to calculate values for the gain coefficient that are in good agreement with experiment.

2–2 INTERACTION OF AN ATOM WITH A RADIATION FIELD

Consider an atom with two nondegenerate energy levels, denoted by a and b. The wave function for the atom can be expanded in terms of the (normalized) energy eigenfunctions of the atom as

$$\psi = a\psi_a + b\psi_b \tag{2-1}$$

The probability of the atom having energy E_a or E_b is then given by

$$P(E_a) = a^*a \tag{2-2}$$

or

$$P(E_b) = b^*b \tag{2-3}$$

If the atom is known to be in a state ψ_a, and if it is completely isolated,[2] the atom will always remain in the state ψ_a. On the other hand, if the atom is in a radiation field specified by an electric intensity $\vec{E}(t)$, it will not be isolated; there will be an interaction energy between the atom and the field

$$V_{\text{int}} = -\vec{p}\cdot\vec{E}(t) \tag{2-4}$$

where $\vec{p}$ is the electric dipole moment of the atom. In this case, the total hamiltonian for the atom is given by

$$H = H_{\text{atom}} + V_{\text{int}} \tag{2-5}$$

and the wave function for the atom develops in time according to the Schroedinger equation

$$H\psi = i\hbar\,\frac{\partial\psi}{\partial t} \tag{2-6}$$

If the magnitude of the interaction energy is small, it is still meaningful to consider an expansion of the wave function ψ in terms of the eigenfunctions

---

[2] Spontaneous emission will be neglected for the moment.

of the atomic hamiltonian. The result of the coupling between the field and the atom is to make the expansion coefficients a and b in Eq. (2-1) functions of time. Inserting (2-5) and (2-1) in the Schroedinger equation, we find that

$$(H_{\text{atom}} + V_{\text{int}})(a\psi_a + b\psi_b) = i\hbar \frac{\partial}{\partial t}(a\psi_a + b\psi_b) \tag{2-7}$$

or

$$aE_a\psi_a + bE_b\psi_b + aV_{\text{int}}\psi_a + bV_{\text{int}}\psi_b = i\hbar\dot{a}\psi_a + i\hbar\dot{b}\psi_b \tag{2-8}$$

Forming the scalar products of this equation with ψ_a and ψ_b and using the orthonormality of ψ_a and ψ_b, we find that the expansion coefficients a and b vary in time according to[3]

$$i\hbar\dot{a} = E_a a + \langle\psi_a|V_{\text{int}}|\psi_b\rangle b - i\hbar a\frac{\gamma_a}{2} \tag{2-9}$$

$$i\hbar\dot{b} = \langle\psi_a|V_{\text{int}}|\psi_b\rangle a + E_b b - i\hbar b\frac{\gamma_b}{2} \tag{2-10}$$

where the decay rates γ_a and γ_b are introduced to account for the fact that in the absence of a radiation field the state of the atom will decay by spontaneous emission. Using Eq. (2-4), we have

$$i\hbar\dot{a} = E_a a - \mu E(t)b - i\hbar a\frac{\gamma_a}{2} \tag{2-11}$$

$$i\hbar\dot{b} = -\mu E(t)a + E_b b - i\hbar b\frac{\gamma_b}{2} \tag{2-12}$$

where

$$\mu = \langle\psi_a|p|\psi_b\rangle \tag{2-13}$$

is called the "matrix element" for the dipole moment of the atom,[4] between states a and b. The expectation value for the dipole moment is

$$\langle\mu\rangle = \langle\psi|p|\psi\rangle \tag{2-14}$$

---

[3] The Dirac symbol $\langle||\rangle$ is used merely as a convenient notation. Thus,

$$\langle\psi_a|V_{\text{int}}|\psi_b\rangle = \int \psi_a^* V_{\text{int}}\psi_b d^N q$$

[4] In our discussion it is assumed that $\vec{p}$ is real, so that $\langle\psi_a|p|\psi_b\rangle = \langle\psi_b|p|\psi_a\rangle$; also, it is assumed that $\vec{p}$ is parallel to $\vec{E}(t)$, so that we can write $\vec{p}\cdot\vec{E}(t) = pE(t)$.

Inserting Eq. (2-1) in (2-14), we find that

$$\langle \mu \rangle = a^*a\langle \psi_a | p | \psi_a \rangle + b^*b\langle \psi_b | p | \psi_b \rangle + a^*b\langle \psi_a | p | \psi_b \rangle + ab^*\langle \psi_b | p | \psi_a \rangle$$

$$(2\text{-}15)$$

Now the terms $\langle \psi_a | p | \psi_a \rangle$ and $\langle \psi_b | p | \psi_b \rangle$ vanish; an atom which is known to be in an energy eigenstate cannot have a radiative dipole moment. Then, from Eq. (2-15), we have

$$\langle \mu \rangle = \mu(a^*b + b^*a) \qquad (2\text{-}16)$$

Equations (2-11) and (2-12) can be interpreted as the equations of motion for the state of the atom. The properties of the atom that concern us here are the probabilities $|a|^2$ and $|b|^2$ and the expectation value of the dipole moment. Rather than solve Eqs. (2-11) and (2-12), it is algebraically simpler to solve for the quantities $|a|^2$, $|b|^2$, a^*b, and ab^* directly. Using (2-11) and (2-12), we obtain

$$\frac{d}{dt}|a|^2 = -\gamma_a|a|^2 + i\frac{\mu E(t)}{\hbar}(a^*b - ab^*) \qquad (2\text{-}17)$$

$$\frac{d}{dt}|b|^2 = -\gamma_b|b|^2 - i\frac{\mu E(t)}{\hbar}(a^*b - ab^*) \qquad (2\text{-}18)$$

$$\frac{d}{dt}(ab^*) = -(i\omega_0 + \gamma)ab^* - i\frac{\mu E(t)}{\hbar}(|a|^2 - |b|^2) \qquad (2\text{-}19)$$

and

$$a^*b = (ab^*)^* \qquad (2\text{-}20)$$

where

$$\omega_0 = \frac{E_a - E_b}{\hbar} \qquad (2\text{-}21)$$

and

$$\gamma = \frac{\gamma_a + \gamma_b}{2} \qquad (2\text{-}22)$$

2–3 DENSITY MATRIX

In our discussion so far, we have considered the interaction between a single atom and a radiation field. In any physical situation, the average behavior of a large number of atoms must be considered. For example, suppose we have a gas containing N atoms per unit volume. According to Eq. (2-16), the expectation value of the dipole moment for the nth atom is

$$\langle \mu \rangle_n = \mu(a_n^* b_n + a_n b_n^*) \qquad (2\text{-}23)$$

Now, because of the statistical nature of the a_k and b_k, different atoms have different dipole moments. However, an "average" atom has a dipole moment

$$\langle \bar{\mu} \rangle = \frac{1}{N} \sum_{n=1}^{N} \mu(a_n^* b_n + a_n b_n^*) \qquad (2\text{-}24)$$

so that the average dipole moment per unit volume can be expressed as

$$N\langle \bar{\mu} \rangle = N\mu(\overline{a^* b} + \overline{ab^*}) \qquad (2\text{-}25)$$

where

$$\overline{a^* b} \equiv \frac{1}{N} \sum_{n=1}^{N} a_n^* b_n \qquad (2\text{-}26)$$

$$\overline{ab^*} \equiv \frac{1}{N} \sum_{n=1}^{N} a_n b_n^* \qquad (2\text{-}27)$$

The quantities $\overline{a^* a}$ and $\overline{b^* b}$ are defined in a similar manner.

It is convenient to express the four quantities $\overline{a^* a}$, $\overline{b^* b}$, $\overline{a^* b}$, and $\overline{ab^*}$ as a matrix, called the "density matrix," whose elements are given by[5]

$$\rho = \begin{bmatrix} \rho_{aa} & \rho_{ab} \\ \rho_{ba} & \rho_{bb} \end{bmatrix} = \begin{bmatrix} \overline{a^* a} & \overline{ab^*} \\ \overline{a^* b} & \overline{b^* b} \end{bmatrix} \qquad (2\text{-}28)$$

Using this notation, we can express the four equations (2-17) through (2-20) as a single matrix equation

$$\dot{\rho} = -i(H\rho - \rho H) - \tfrac{1}{2}(\Gamma\rho + \rho\Gamma) \qquad (2\text{-}29)$$

---

[5] The matrix that we call a density matrix might more properly be called a "reduced" density matrix. We have explicitly assumed that the atoms under consideration have only two energy levels, but by introducing the decay constants γ_a and γ_b, we have implicitly assumed that the atoms have other energy levels. In a more formal treatment, the density matrix would take into account all the states of the atoms; in the present discussion, this would result in unnecessary complication. We may note, however, that some of the properties of the "full" density matrix are not possessed by the reduced density matrix, for example, the trace of the reduced density matrix is not conserved.

where $\mathbf{H}$ is the hamiltonian matrix

$$\mathbf{H} = \begin{bmatrix} E_a & V_{\text{int}} \\ V_{\text{int}} & E_b \end{bmatrix} \tag{2-30}$$

and $\boldsymbol{\Gamma}$ is the decay matrix

$$\boldsymbol{\Gamma} = \begin{bmatrix} \gamma_a & 0 \\ 0 & \gamma_b \end{bmatrix} \tag{2-31}$$

The density matrix defined by Eq. (2-28) provides a very convenient formalism for solving problems involving quantum-mechanical systems. In the present situation, we consider the density matrix for a class of atoms that are excited to state a at time t_0. We denote the density matrix for such a system by $\rho(a,t,t_0)$. Since the class was known to be in state a at time t_0, we have as an initial condition

$$\rho(a,t_0,t_0) = \begin{bmatrix} 1 & 0 \\ 0 & 0 \end{bmatrix} \tag{2-32}$$

As time progresses, the density matrix will evolve according to Eq. (2-29).

To determine the properties of the quantum-mechanical system at some later time t, we must find the density matrix $\rho(a,t)$ corresponding to the addition of all the "elementary" density matrices $\rho(a,t,t_{0i})$. That is, for each "class" of atoms excited to state a at a time $t_{0i} < t$, there will be a density matrix $\rho(a,t,t_{0i})$; to determine the overall behavior of the system at some later time t, we must consider the contributions from all these "classes" of atoms. Suppose that atoms are excited to state a at a constant rate λ_a. The density matrix $\rho(a,t)$ describing the overall response of the system at time t is then given by

$$\rho(a,t) = \int_{-\infty}^{t} \lambda_a \rho(a,t,t_0)\, dt_0 \tag{2-33}$$

If we differentiate this equation, we find, using the initial condition (2-32), that

$$\dot{\rho}(a,t) = \lambda_a + \int_{-\infty}^{t} \lambda_a \dot{\rho}(a,t,t_0)\, dt_0 \tag{2-34}$$

which, upon introducing (2-29) for $\dot{\rho}(a,t,t_0)$, becomes

$$\dot{\rho}(a,t) = \lambda_a - \int_{-\infty}^{t} \lambda_a [i(\mathbf{H}\rho - \rho\mathbf{H}) + \tfrac{1}{2}(\boldsymbol{\Gamma}\rho + \rho\boldsymbol{\Gamma})]\, dt_0 \tag{2-35}$$

where we have omitted the arguments (a,t,t_0) on the right-hand side for brevity.

If we assume that H does not depend on t_0, using Eq. (2-33), we find that (2-35) can be integrated to yield

$$\dot{\rho}(a,t) = \lambda_a - i[H\rho(a,t) - \rho(a,t)H] - \tfrac{1}{2}[\Gamma\rho(a,t) + \rho(a,t)\Gamma] \quad (2\text{-}36)$$

The above procedure could be repeated for atoms that are excited to state b at time t_0, in which case we would obtain an equation analogous to (2-36) for $\rho(b,t)$. If both states a and b are being excited, the overall response of the system at time t will be described by the density matrix

$$\rho(t) = \sum_{\alpha = a,b} \rho(\alpha,t) \quad (2\text{-}37)$$

The "complete" density matrix $\rho(t)$, henceforth to be called simply the "density matrix," will obey an equation of motion

$$\dot{\rho} = \lambda - i(H\rho - \rho H) - \tfrac{1}{2}(\Gamma\rho + \rho\Gamma) \quad (2\text{-}38)$$

where λ is the excitation matrix

$$\lambda = \begin{bmatrix} \lambda_a & 0 \\ 0 & \lambda_b \end{bmatrix} \quad (2\text{-}39)$$

Except for the term λ, Eq. (2-38) looks identical to (2-29). It should be remembered, however, that the density matrices satisfying the two equations are quite different. The density matrix $\rho(t)$ which satisfies Eq. (2-38) represents the ensemble average at time t for *all* atoms excited to states a or b at $t_0 < t$, whereas the elementary density matrix $\rho(a,t,t_0)$ which satisfies (2-29) represents only an ensemble of atoms excited to state a at time t_0.

The density matrix $\rho(t)$ is, of course, the more useful of the two density matrices discussed above, for it enables us to solve problems without resorting to an integration over excitation time t_0. We should stress, however, that the equation of motion (2-38) for the density matrix $\rho(t)$ was derived with the assumption that the hamiltonian for the system was independent of t_0. If this is not the case, then we must use equations like (2-35) and (2-37) to find the density matrix, rather than (2-38).

In this chapter, we shall consider systems for which the hamiltonian is independent of t_0. The equations of motion for the elements of the density matrix are then found by expanding Eq. (2-38):

$$\dot{\rho}_{aa} = \lambda_a - \gamma_a \rho_{aa} + i \frac{\mu E(t)}{\hbar} (\rho_{ba} - \rho_{ab}) \qquad (2\text{-}40)$$

$$\dot{\rho}_{bb} = \lambda_b - \gamma_b \rho_{bb} - i \frac{\mu E(t)}{\hbar} (\rho_{ba} - \rho_{ab}) \qquad (2\text{-}41)$$

$$\dot{\rho}_{ab} = -(i\omega_0 + \gamma)\rho_{ab} - i \frac{\mu E(t)}{\hbar} (\rho_{aa} - \rho_{bb}) \qquad (2\text{-}42)$$

$$\rho_{ba} = \rho_{ab}^* \qquad (2\text{-}43)$$

2–4 RATE–EQUATION APPROXIMATION

Some insight into the general nature of the solutions of Eqs. (2-40) through (2-43) can be gained from considering the direct integration of (2-42). Using standard techniques, we obtain

$$\rho_{ab} = -i \frac{e^{(i\omega_0 + \gamma)t}}{\hbar} \int (\rho_{aa} - \rho_{bb})\mu E(t) e^{-(i\omega_0 + \gamma)t} \, dt \qquad (2\text{-}44)$$

If the factor $\rho_{aa} - \rho_{bb}$ is not a function of time, then it can be taken outside the integral. Equation (2-44) and its complex conjugate can then be inserted in (2-40) and (2-41) to yield equations for $\dot{\rho}_{aa}$ and $\dot{\rho}_{bb}$ in terms of constants times ρ_{aa} and ρ_{bb}. The resultant equations, which are called rate equations, are very useful for describing the general interactions between radiation and matter. The rate-equation approximation to Eqs. (2-40) and (2-41) is valid in two principal situations.[6]

The first situation occurs when $E(t)$ is small in magnitude. This is the situation encountered in the ordinary incoherent emission and absorption of light. The integral in this case will be small, and examination of Eqs. (2-40) and (2-41) shows that $\rho_{aa} - \rho_{bb}$ is approximately constant in time.

The second situation occurs when $E(t)$ is a monochromatic function of time. We shall consider this case in some detail. Suppose that

$$E(t) = E_0 \cos \omega t \qquad (2\text{-}45)$$

---

[6] When the rate-equation approximation is not valid, the interpretation of $\rho(t)$ as a complete density matrix of the type described in the preceding section also is not valid, and we must revert to consideration of the elementary density matrices $\rho(t, t_0)$, which obey Eq. (2-29).

where E_0 is a constant. Assuming, for the moment, that the rate-equation approximation is indeed valid, from Eq. (2-44) we find that

$$\rho_{ab} = -i\frac{\mu E_0}{2\hbar}(\rho_{aa} - \rho_{bb})e^{(i\omega_0 + \gamma)t} \int e^{[i(\omega - \omega_0) - \gamma]t}\, dt \qquad (2\text{-}46)$$

where we neglect the integral of the term which oscillates at $(\omega_0 + \omega)$. Carrying out the integration, we obtain

$$\rho_{ab} = i\frac{\mu E_0}{2\hbar}(\rho_{aa} - \rho_{bb})\frac{e^{i\omega t}}{i(\omega - \omega_0) + \gamma} \qquad (2\text{-}47)$$

Using this equation, together with (2-43), in Eqs. (2-40) and (2-41), we find after some algebra that

$$\dot{\rho}_{aa} = \lambda_a - \gamma_a\rho_{aa} - \frac{\mu^2 E_0^2}{\hbar^2}\left[\frac{\gamma}{(\omega - \omega_0)^2 + \gamma^2}\right](\rho_{aa} - \rho_{bb}) \qquad (2\text{-}48)$$

$$\dot{\rho}_{bb} = \lambda_b - \gamma_b\rho_{bb} + \frac{\mu^2 E_0^2}{\hbar^2}\left[\frac{\gamma}{(\omega - \omega_0)^2 + \gamma^2}\right](\rho_{aa} - \rho_{bb}) \qquad (2\text{-}49)$$

In taking the factor $\rho_{aa} - \rho_{bb}$ outside the integral in Eq. (2-46), we tacitly assumed that $\dot{\rho}_{aa} - \dot{\rho}_{bb} = 0$. By setting the left-hand sides of Eqs. (2-48) and (2-49) equal to zero, we see that this assumption requires that

$$\rho_{aa} - \rho_{bb} = \frac{\lambda_a/\gamma_a - \lambda_b/\gamma_b}{1 + \dfrac{\gamma^2\mu^2 E_0^2}{\gamma_a\gamma_b\hbar^2[(\omega - \omega_0)^2 + \gamma^2]}} \qquad (2\text{-}50)$$

The notation in the preceding equations can be simplified by noting that in a gas with a density of N atoms per unit volume, the average number of atoms per unit volume in state a is $n_a = N\rho_{aa}$; and similarly, $n_b = N\rho_{bb}$. We can also define quantities called "excitation rates" by $\Lambda_a = N\lambda_a$ and $\Lambda_b = N\lambda_b$. The excitation rates Λ_a and Λ_b thus represent the number of atoms per unit volume excited to state a or b per unit time. The rate equations (2-48) and (2-49) then become

$$\dot{n}_a = \Lambda_a - \gamma_a n_a - R(n_a - n_b) \qquad (2\text{-}51)$$

$$\dot{n}_b = \Lambda_b - \gamma_b n_b + R(n_a - n_b) \qquad (2\text{-}52)$$

where

$$R = \frac{\mu^2 E_0^2}{\hbar^2}\left[\frac{\gamma}{(\omega - \omega_0)^2 + \gamma^2}\right] \qquad (2\text{-}53)$$

is called the "rate constant." Equation (2-50) may then be written as

$$n_a - n_b = \frac{\mathscr{I}_0}{1 + (\gamma/\gamma_a\gamma_b)R} \tag{2-54}$$

where

$$\mathscr{I}_0 = \frac{\Lambda_a}{\gamma_a} - \frac{\Lambda_b}{\gamma_b} \tag{2-55}$$

is called the "inversion density." From Eq. (2-54) we see that $\mathscr{I}_0$ is the number of atoms per unit volume in state a less the number of atoms per unit volume in state b, in the absence of a field.

The rate equations (2-51) and (2-52) illustrate the general nature of the solution of the equations of motion for the density matrix. The first term on the right side of Eq. (2-51) represents the increase in the population due to excitation; the second term gives the decrease in population due to spontaneous emission; the last term describes the effects of stimulated emission or absorption (depending on the sign of $n_a - n_b$) on the population of state a.

2–5 DISPERSION THEORY

We shall now consider the problem of determining the gain coefficient and refractive index of a gas. In this section, we shall assume that all the gas atoms are stationary. Although this is obviously a poor approximation to the actual physical situation in a real gas, it is pedagogically desirable to consider the simplest case first; in the next section we shall see how our results are modified when thermal motion of the gas atoms is considered.

We consider the radiation field at a certain point in the gas to be a monochromatic scalar function of time

$$E(t) = E_0 \cos \omega t \tag{2-56}$$

As shown in the preceding section, the rate-equation approximation is valid in this case. In order to determine the gain coefficient and refractive index of the gas, we first determine the polarization $P(t)$ of the gas under the influence of the field $E(t)$. The ratio of the polarization to the field determines the susceptibility of the gas; and once the susceptibility is known, we can find the gain coefficient g_l and the refractive index n by the relations

$$g_l = -\frac{\omega}{c}\chi'' \tag{2-57}$$

$$n = 1 + \tfrac{1}{2}\chi' \tag{2-58}$$

where χ' and χ'' are the real and imaginary parts of the complex susceptibility.[7]
The magnitude of the polarization of the gas is given by

$$P(t) = N\mu(\rho_{ab} + \rho_{ab}^*) \tag{2-59}$$

For monochromatic excitation, we have already seen in Eq. (2-47) that

$$\rho_{ab} = i\frac{\mu E_0}{2\hbar}(n_a - n_b)\frac{e^{i\omega t}}{i(\omega - \omega_0) + \gamma} \tag{2-60}$$

If we use this result in Eq. (2-59), we find that

$$P(t) = \frac{\mu^2 E_0(n_a - n_b)}{\hbar}\left[\frac{(\omega - \omega_0)\cos\omega t - \gamma\sin\omega t}{(\omega - \omega_0)^2 + \gamma^2}\right] \tag{2-61}$$

Now, according to Eq. (2-54),

$$n_a - n_b = \frac{\mathscr{I}_0}{1 + \dfrac{\gamma^2\mu^2 E_0^2}{\gamma_a\gamma_b\hbar^2[(\omega - \omega_0)^2 + \gamma^2]}} \tag{2-62}$$

Inserting this result in Eq. (2-61), we obtain for the polarization

$$P(t) = \frac{\mu^2 E_0\mathscr{I}_0}{\hbar}\left[\frac{(\omega - \omega_0)\cos\omega t - \gamma\sin\omega t}{(\omega - \omega_0)^2 + \gamma^2[1 + (\mu^2 E_0^2/\gamma_a\gamma_b\hbar^2)]}\right] \tag{2-63}$$

This equation can be written in a somewhat neater form by defining a saturated
decay rate

$$\gamma_s = \gamma\left(1 + \frac{W}{W_{s0}}\right)^{\frac{1}{2}} \tag{2-64}$$

where

$$W = \frac{c\epsilon_0}{2}E_0^2 \tag{2-65}$$

is the intensity in the field at the point under consideration,[8] and

$$W_{s0} = \frac{\gamma_a\gamma_b\hbar^2\epsilon_0 c}{2\mu^2} \tag{2-66}$$

[7] The relations between the various macroscopic parameters of a material are discussed
in Appendix 1.
[8] See Appendix 1.

is called the "saturation parameter" for the gas. We then have for the polarization that

$$P(t) = \frac{\mu^2 E_0 \mathscr{I}_0}{\hbar} \left[\frac{(\omega - \omega_0) \cos \omega t - \gamma \sin \omega t}{(\omega - \omega_0)^2 + {\gamma_s}^2} \right] \tag{2-67}$$

or

$$P(t) = \epsilon_0 E_0 (\chi' \cos \omega t + \chi'' \sin \omega t) \tag{2-68}$$

where

$$\chi' = \frac{\mu^2 \mathscr{I}_0}{\epsilon_0 \hbar} \left[\frac{\omega - \omega_0}{(\omega - \omega_0)^2 + {\gamma_s}^2} \right] \tag{2-69}$$

and

$$\chi'' = -\frac{\mu^2 \mathscr{I}_0}{\epsilon_0 \hbar} \left[\frac{\gamma}{(\omega - \omega_0)^2 + {\gamma_s}^2} \right] \tag{2-70}$$

are the real and imaginary parts of the complex susceptibility.

By using these last equations in (2-57) and (2-58), we obtain the gain coefficient and refractive index as

$$g_l(\omega) = \frac{\omega \mu^2 \mathscr{I}_0}{c \epsilon_0 \hbar} \left[\frac{\gamma}{(\omega - \omega_0)^2 + {\gamma_s}^2} \right] \tag{2-71}$$

and

$$n(\omega) = 1 + \frac{\mu^2 \mathscr{I}_0}{2 \epsilon_0 \hbar} \left[\frac{\omega - \omega_0}{(\omega - \omega_0)^2 + {\gamma_s}^2} \right] \tag{2-72}$$

2–6 LINE BROADENING

In any real gas, the atoms are in continuous motion because of thermal agitation. The thermal motion of the atoms causes an increase in the linewidth of radiation emitted or absorbed by the gas. This line broadening is primarily of two types: "collision broadening" and "Doppler broadening." Collision broadening (sometimes called "pressure broadening") is caused by the fact that the randomly moving gas atoms will occasionally "collide." Doppler broadening is caused by the fact that the apparent frequency of radiation emitted by a moving atom will be Doppler-shifted toward higher or lower frequencies, depending on whether the motion of the atom is toward or away from the observer.

Collision broadening and Doppler broadening are fundamentally different in nature. The principal effect of collision broadening is to shorten the effective decay time for radiation emitted by an atom. This effect is the same for all the atoms in the gas; hence collision broadening is a form of what is called "homogeneous" broadening. (Notice that the "natural" line broadening defined by the spontaneous decay rates γ_a and γ_b is also a form of homogeneous broadening.) On the other hand, Doppler broadening is caused by the superposition of the Doppler-shifted radiation emitted by different atoms in the gas. In the limit where natural broadening and collision broadening could be neglected, each atom would emit a well-defined frequency, but Doppler broadening would still be present because of the different apparent frequencies emitted by different atoms. Broadening of this type is called "inhomogeneous" broadening.

In this section we shall consider how collision and Doppler broadening affect the interaction of radiation and matter. A complete description of line broadening in real gases would be hopelessly complicated by the large number of possible interactions between different atoms in a gas. Nevertheless, by considering only the dominant interactions, we can modify the theory phenomenologically so that it is in good agreement with experiment. We shall begin by considering collision broadening.

We should note at the outset that in the present context the term "collision" does not refer to a collision in the sense of classical mechanics. An optical collision occurs whenever two atoms come close enough together so that they cause noticeable effects on each other.[9] The collision process is often described by a perturbation energy which depends on the distance between two atoms. The effective range of the perturbation energy defines an "optical-collision cross section," which is simply the area of a circle whose radius is equal to the effective range of the perturbation energy. In practice, the exact form of the perturbation energy is not usually known, and optical-collision cross sections are usually measured experimentally.

In general, the collisional perturbation energy between two atoms will decrease smoothly as the distance between the atoms increases, and it is not immediately clear how to define the "effective" range of the perturbation energy. Some insight into this problem can be gained by considering the general nature of collision broadening.

The most useful model for *visualization* is the classical model, where we imagine that the emission of light by an atom occurs by a gradual decay in the energy of the atom over a time interval approximately equal to γ^{-1}. If no collision occurs during the time interval γ^{-1}, then the radiation emitted by the atom will be sinusoidal during the emission interval. However, if a

---

[9] In our present discussion the effects of "three-body" collisions are neglected. This is a good approximation at low pressures.

collision occurs during the emission, the phase of the radiation will be altered during the time of the collision.[10].

Two types of collisions can be distinguished, depending on the magnitude of the phase shift during the collision. The first type, called a "hard" collision, occurs when the phase of the radiation at the end of the collision is many cycles different from what it would have been if the collision had not occurred. This type of collision has the effect of completely disrupting the phase of the emission; the phase of the radiation after the collision has no correlation with the phase before the emission, and the emission appears to have a reduced lifetime. In the second type, called a "soft" collision, the phase of the radiation at the end of the emission is only slightly different from what it would have been if the collision had not occurred. This type of collision cannot formally be accounted for by simply decreasing the effective lifetime of the atom.

The effects of hard collisions are comparatively easy to treat theoretically; they simply give rise to a collisional decay rate which is approximately proportional to the gas pressure. The effects of soft collisions, however, are more complicated.[11] We shall assume that the effects of collision broadening can be accounted for in our discussion of the preceding three sections by simply replacing γ in the equations of motion for the density matrix [see Eq. (2-42)] by a decay rate γ', which includes the effects of collisions:

$$\gamma' = \gamma + (\text{constant} \times \text{pressure}) \qquad (2\text{-}73)$$

The analysis then proceeds in the same manner as before. We obtain for the gain coefficient and refractive index of a gas, including collision broadening,

$$g_i(\omega) = \frac{\omega \mu^2 \mathscr{I}_0}{c \epsilon_0 \hbar} \left[\frac{\gamma'}{(\omega - \omega_0)^2 + \gamma_s'^2} \right] \qquad (2\text{-}74)$$

$$n(\omega) = 1 + \frac{\mu^2 \mathscr{I}_0}{2 \epsilon_0 \hbar} \left[\frac{\omega - \omega_0}{(\omega - \omega_0)^2 + \gamma_s'^2} \right] \qquad (2\text{-}75)$$

where

$$\gamma_s' = \gamma' \left(1 + \frac{W}{W_{s0}} \right)^{1/2} \qquad (2\text{-}76)$$

[10] A more complete treatment of collisions would consider changes in the trajectory of the atom, in addition to the frequency shifts that are considered here.

[11] In general, soft collisions give rise to a different functional form for the line shape.

and the saturation parameter becomes

$$W_{s0} = \frac{\gamma_a \gamma_b \hbar^2 \epsilon_0 c}{2\mu^2} \frac{\gamma'}{\gamma} \qquad (2\text{-}77)$$

Notice that we have used the same symbol for the collision-broadened saturation parameter as for the natural-broadened saturation parameter. Inasmuch as we shall have no further use for the natural-broadened saturation parameter, this should cause no problem.

We now turn to consideration of Doppler broadening. In order to determine the line broadening caused by the Doppler effect, it is necessary, of course, to know the distribution of velocities of the atoms in the gas. We shall assume that the distribution of velocities follows the Maxwell-Boltzmann distribution law,[12] so that the probability of an atom having a velocity whose z component lies between v_z and $(v_z + dv_z)$ is

$$P(v_z)\, dv_z = \sqrt{\frac{2M}{\pi kT}}\, e^{-[Mv_z{}^2/2kT]}\, dv_z \qquad (2\text{-}78)$$

where M is the mass of the atom, T is the temperature, and k is Boltzmann's constant.

According to the standard Doppler-shift formula, the apparent frequency ω' of radiation from an atom moving with a velocity v_z in the direction of a stationary observer is

$$\omega' = \omega_0\left(1 + \frac{v_z}{c}\right) \qquad (2\text{-}79)$$

where ω_0 is the frequency that would be observed if the atom were at rest. By combining this equation with (2-78), we find that the probability that an atom has a Doppler-shifted resonance frequency between ω' and $(\omega' + d\omega')$ is given by

$$P(\omega')\, d\omega' = \frac{2}{\sqrt{\pi}\, \Delta\omega_D}\, e^{-[(\omega' - \omega_0)/\Delta\omega_D]^2}\, d\omega' \qquad (2\text{-}80)$$

where

$$\Delta\omega_D = \omega_0\sqrt{\frac{2kT}{Mc^2}} \qquad (2\text{-}81)$$

---

[12] It should be stressed that this is an assumption, which is not always valid when applied to gas discharges. Nevertheless, experimental measurements of line profiles indicate that it is a good approximation for most lines.

Note that $\Delta\omega_D$ represents the half-width of the line at the $1/e$ intensity point. It is conventional to quote numerical values of the Doppler width by giving the full-width at half-maximum intensity. $\Delta\omega_D$ is related to the conventional Doppler width by

$$\Delta\omega_D = \frac{\text{Doppler width, Hz}}{4\pi\sqrt{\ln 2}} \tag{2-82}$$

We can now determine the gain coefficient and refractive index of a gas, including the effects of both collision and Doppler broadening. The contribution to the gain coefficient at a frequency ω by atoms whose Doppler-shifted frequency is ω' is given by Eq. (2-74), with ω' substituted for ω_0. On the other hand, the probability of the atom having a Doppler-shifted frequency ω' is given by Eq. (2-80). The total gain coefficient at a frequency Ω is thus found by multiplying Eq. (2-74) by the probability distribution function (2-80) and integrating over all frequencies $0 \le \omega' \le \infty$, so that

$$g_l(\omega) = \frac{g_{l0}\gamma'}{\pi} \int_0^\infty \frac{e^{-[(\omega'-\omega_0)/\Delta\omega_D]^2}}{(\omega-\omega')^2 + \gamma_s'^2}\, d\omega' \tag{2-83}$$

where

$$g_{l0} = \frac{\sqrt{\pi}\,\omega\mu^2\mathscr{I}_0}{c\epsilon_0\hbar\,\Delta\omega_D} \tag{2-84}$$

The refractive index is found by using the same reasoning. We have

$$n(\omega) = 1 + \frac{g_{l0}c}{2\pi\omega} \int_0^\infty \frac{(\omega-\omega')\,e^{-[(\omega'-\omega_0)/\Delta\omega_D]^2}}{(\omega-\omega')^2 + \gamma_s'^2}\, d\omega' \tag{2-85}$$

The above integrals can be written in neater form by defining a new integration variable

$$t = \frac{\omega' - \omega_0}{\Delta\omega_D} \tag{2-86}$$

If we further define a "normalized frequency"

$$\xi = \frac{\omega - \omega_0}{\Delta\omega_D} \tag{2-87}$$

and a "broadening parameter"

$$\eta = \frac{\gamma_s'}{\Delta\omega_D} \tag{2-88}$$

we can rewrite Eqs. (2-83) and (2-85) as

$$g_l(\omega) = \frac{g_{l0}\gamma'}{\pi\gamma_s'} \int_{-\infty}^{\infty} \frac{\eta e^{-t^2}}{(\xi - t)^2 + \eta^2} \, dt \tag{2-89}$$

and

$$n(\omega) = 1 + \frac{g_{l0}c}{2\pi\omega} \int_{-\infty}^{\infty} \frac{(\xi - t)e^{-t^2}}{(\xi - t)^2 + \eta^2} \, dt \tag{2-90}$$

where we have made use of the fact that $\Delta\omega_D \ll \omega_0$ to replace the lower integration limit $-\omega_0/\Delta\omega_D$ in these equations by $-\infty$.

The integrals in Eqs. (2-90) and (2-89) define the real and imaginary parts of a complex function called the "plasma dispersion function":[13]

$$Z(\xi + i\eta) = Z_r(\xi + i\eta) + iZ_i(\xi + i\eta) \tag{2-91}$$

Figure 2-1 shows the general behavior of this function. In terms of the plasma dispersion function, we have

$$g_l(\omega) = \frac{g_{l0}}{\sqrt{\pi}\,[1 + (W/W_{s0})]^{1/2}} Z_i(\xi + i\eta) \tag{2-92}$$

$$n(\omega) = 1 - \frac{g_{l0}c}{2\sqrt{\pi}\,\omega} Z_r(\xi + i\eta) \tag{2-93}$$

These last equations are the basic result of our analysis in this chapter.

We may note from the relation $Z(0) = i\sqrt{\pi}$ that the constant g_{l0} defined in Eq. (2-84) has a simple physical significance: it is the gain coefficient at ω_0 in the limit where the broadening parameter is negligible and there is no saturation.

It is instructive to consider the limiting behavior of the plasma dispersion function in two cases. The first case of interest occurs if we assume that the broadening parameter η is negligible, that is, $\gamma_s' \ll \Delta\omega_D$. A spectral line having this property is known as an "inhomogeneous line." In this case, we have

$$Z(\xi) = -2e^{-\xi^2} \int_0^{\xi} e^{t^2} \, dt + i\sqrt{\pi}\, e^{-\xi^2} \tag{2-94}$$

so that the gain coefficient is

$$g_l(\omega) = \frac{g_{l0}}{[1 + (W/W_{s0})]^{1/2}} e^{-[(\omega - \omega_0)/\Delta\omega_0]^2} \tag{2-95}$$

[13] A discussion of the plasma dispersion function will be found in Appendix 2.

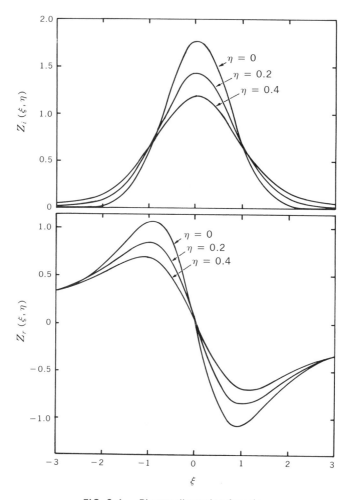

FIG. 2-1.   Plasma dispersion function.

and the refractive index is

$$n(\omega) = 1 + \frac{g_{lo}c}{\sqrt{\pi}\,\omega} e^{-[(\omega-\omega_0)/\Delta\omega_D]^2} \int_0^{(\omega-\omega_0)/\Delta\omega_D} e^{t^2}\,dt \qquad (2\text{-}96)$$

The other case of interest occurs when the broadening parameter η is very large, that is, $\gamma_s' \gg \Delta\omega_D$. A spectral line having this property is known as a "homogeneous line." In this case, we have

$$Z(\xi + i\eta) \xrightarrow[\eta \to \infty]{} -\frac{1}{\xi + i\eta} \qquad (2\text{-}97)$$

so that the gain coefficient is given by

$$g_l(\omega) = \frac{\Delta\omega_D g_{l0}}{\sqrt{\pi}} \frac{\gamma'}{(\omega - \omega_0)^2 + \gamma_s'^2} \tag{2-98}$$

and the refractive index is given by

$$n(\omega) = 1 + \frac{cg_{l0} \Delta\omega_D}{2\omega\sqrt{\pi}} \frac{\omega - \omega_0}{(\omega - \omega_0)^2 + \gamma_s'^2} \tag{2-99}$$

It is interesting to note the saturation behavior of the gain coefficient. At $\omega = \omega_0$, we have in general [see Eq. (2-92)] that

$$g_l(\omega_0) = \frac{g_{l0}}{\sqrt{\pi}\,[1 + (W/W_{s0})]^{\frac{1}{2}}} Z_i\{i\gamma'[1 + (W/W_{s0})]^{\frac{1}{2}}\} \tag{2-100}$$

For an inhomogeneous line, this reduces to [see Eq. (2-95)]

$$g_l(\omega_0) = \frac{g_{l0}}{[1 + (W/W_{s0})]^{\frac{1}{2}}} \tag{2-101}$$

whereas for a homogeneous line, this reduces to [see Eq. (2-98]

$$g_l(\omega_0) = \frac{\Delta\omega_D}{\sqrt{\pi}\,\gamma'} \frac{g_{l0}}{[1 + (W/W_{s0})]} \tag{2-102}$$

We see from an examination of these equations that the gain coefficient for an inhomogeneous line saturates more slowly than does the gain coefficient for a homogeneous line. This phenomenon has a simple explanation in terms of a concept known as "hole burning."

The concept of hole burning comes from the consideration that any *particular* atom in a gas can "interact" only with radiation whose frequency lies within a range $\sim \pm\gamma_s'$ from the atom's resonance frequency. For a homogeneous line, $\gamma_s' \gg \Delta\omega_D$, so that all the atoms in the gas can interact with radiation having any frequency within the linewidth of the transition. On the other hand, for an inhomogeneous line, $\gamma_s' \ll \Delta\omega_D$, so that only a fraction of the atoms in the gas can interact with radiation of any given frequency within $\Delta\omega_D$. If a strong field at a frequency ω_1 is applied to a gas having an inhomogeneous transition, the population difference $n_a - n_b$ will be "depleted," but *only* for those atoms having Doppler-shifted resonance frequencies in the range $\omega' \approx \omega_1 \pm \gamma_s'$. If we were to make a plot of population difference versus frequency for this situation, it would appear as shown in Figure 2-2. The field at ω_1 is thus said to "burn a hole" in the line. Now the "width" of the hole is proportional to $\gamma_s' = \gamma'[1 + (W/W_{s0})]^{\frac{1}{2}}$, whereas the "depth" of the hole is proportional to $[1 + (W/W_{s0})]^{-1}$. The amount of population depletion, on the other hand, is proportional to the "area" of the hole, which is therefore proportional to $[1 + (W/W_{s0})]^{-\frac{1}{2}}$. Since the gain coefficient is proportional to $n_a - n_b$, the gain coefficient for an inhomogene-

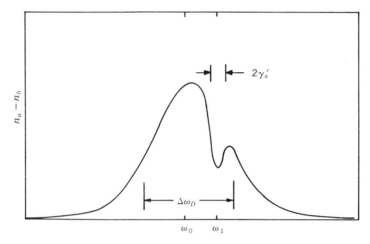

FIG. 2-2.   "Hole" burning.

ous line will saturate as $[1 + (W/W_{s0})]^{-\frac{1}{2}}$. For a homogeneous line, the width of the saturation is simply determined by the total linewidth and is independent of the incident field intensity. A homogeneous line thus saturates as $[1 + (W/W_{s0})]^{-1}$.

Note that γ_s' determines the frequency range over which saturation effects occur and can be considered a linewidth. In fact, all the decay rates γ, γ', and γ_s' can be interpreted as linewidths; we shall call γ the "natural linewidth"; γ' the "homogeneous linewidth"; and γ_s' the "hole width." For example, $\gamma/2\pi$ determines the half-width at half-maximum intensity of a spectral line for which collision-broadening can be neglected.[14]

We conclude this section by noting that there are other sources of line broadening which are often observed experimentally but which have not been

---

[14] When numerical values are given, they are usually quoted in radians per second if the parameter is being considered as a decay rate, and in hertz if the parameter is being considered as a linewidth. Thus,

$$\gamma \text{ (decay rate)} = 2\pi\gamma \text{ (linewidth)}$$

discussed here. It would be impossible to describe all these in detail, but we note that the basic distinction between broadening mechanisms (with respect to effects observed in gas lasers) is whether they give rise to homogeneous or inhomogeneous broadening.

REFERENCES

Most of the references for this chapter are to general physics and optics textbooks. Since the reader undoubtedly has his favorites, we shall not try to persuade him to use others. Two special references are in order, however.

1. R. C. Tolman, "Principles of Statistical Mechanics," p. 325, Oxford University Press (Clarendon), New York, 1938.

Our use of the density matrix is quite well described by Tolman. Many of the later treatments do not give so much physical insight as does his.

2. W. E. Lamb, Jr., in W. E. Brittin and B. W. Downs (eds.), "Lectures in Theoretical Physics," p. 435, Interscience Publishers, Inc., New York, 1960.

Our general approach to determining the optical constants of a gas is described in this reference, although much of the specific discussion is not applicable to our case.

3 LAMB'S THEORY OF GAS LASERS

A comprehensive theoretical description of gas lasers has been developed by Professor W. E. Lamb, Jr. In this chapter, we shall describe Lamb's theory and consider some of its implications. The model of a gas discharge employed in this chapter is the same as that used in Chapter 2. Thus we assume that a population inversion described by an inversion density $\mathscr{I}_0$ [see Eq. (2-55)] is created on a radiative transition between energy levels a and b of an atom and that we need only consider that these levels are associated with decay rates γ_a and γ_b. The transition between levels a and b is described by a "center" frequency ω_0, a natural linewidth γ, a homogeneous linewidth γ', and a Doppler linewidth $\Delta\omega_D$.

The model of a gas laser used in this chapter consists of a gas discharge, placed between two plane-parallel mirrors of equal (high) reflectance r. The mirrors are said to constitute an "optical cavity."

3–1 LASER CAVITIES

The function of the optical cavity in a laser is to provide positive "feedback" of radiation to the gas discharge, which acts as an optical amplifier. If the feedback is sufficiently large, the system as a whole will be regenerative and will function as a light oscillator.

In order for the feedback in the cavity to be positive, the optical path length between the mirrors must be an integer number of half wavelengths. The resonance frequencies of the cavity are thus given by

$$\Omega_n = n\pi \frac{c}{L} \tag{3-1}$$

where n is an integer, c is the phase velocity of light in a vacuum, and L is the "passive" optical length of the cavity. The passive optical length of the cavity includes the "bulk" refractive index of the gas but does not include that part of the refractive index attributable to anomalous dispersion on the laser transition.

Fields in the cavity having frequencies which satisfy the resonance condition (3-1) for different values of n are called different "longitudinal modes" of the cavity. The various field distributions perpendicular to the axis which reproduce themselves after a complete traversal of the cavity are called different "transverse modes." In this chapter, we confine our attention to the so-called "lowest-order" transverse mode, which we assume to be a uniform-amplitude plane wave. We do consider, however, the possibility that several longitudinal modes may be simultaneously excited in the cavity.

An important characteristic of a cavity is the rate at which optical energy decays in the cavity. Several parameters are commonly used to describe this rate. In this chapter, we shall use the "temporal loss coefficient" α_t, which is defined as the fractional intensity loss per unit time. If diffraction loss can be neglected,[1] α_t is determined by the mirror reflectance r and the cavity length L. In particular,

$$\alpha_t = \frac{c}{L}(1 - r) \tag{3-2}$$

We shall assume that α_t does not depend on the frequency of any modes lying within the oscillation bandwidth of a given laser transition.

Another parameter often used to describe the decay of energy in a cavity is the Q (quality factor) of the cavity. The Q of a cavity for the nth longitudinal mode is given by

$$Q_n = \frac{\Omega_n}{\alpha_{tn}} \tag{3-3}$$

3–2 SELF-CONSISTENCY EQUATIONS

The operation of a gas laser can be analyzed by using two different methods: (1) a "wave" analysis and (2) a "mode" analysis. In the wave analysis, the fields in the laser are interpreted as running waves which propagate back and forth between the laser mirrors. In the mode analysis, the fields in the laser are interpreted as standing waves with time-varying amplitudes. The spatial variation of the electric field in the nth longitudinal mode must be

$$U_n(z) = \sin \frac{n\pi}{L} z \tag{3-4}$$

[1] If the radius of the mirrors is much larger than $\sqrt{L\lambda}$, this is a good approximation.

to satisfy the boundary conditions at the laser mirrors, and a general field in the cavity can be expanded in a sum over these longitudinal modes as[2]

$$E(z,t) = \sum_n A_n(t)U_n(z) \tag{3-5}$$

The $A_n(t)$ can be further expanded as

$$A_n(t) = E_n(t) \cos [\omega_n t + \varphi_n(t)] \tag{3-6}$$

where ω_n is a constant, and $E_n(t)$ and $\varphi_n(t)$ are slowly varying functions of time. The quantities of interest in the mode analysis are the mode amplitudes $E_n(t)$ and the mode frequencies[3] $\omega_n + \dot{\varphi}_n$.

The wave analysis and the mode analysis both lead to equivalent results. It is easier, however, to treat the problem of simultaneous oscillation in several longitudinal modes by using the mode analysis, and most of the discussion in this chapter is restricted to this point of view.

In the mode analysis, the amplification of the nth longitudinal mode is described by the "temporal gain coefficient" g_{tn}, which is related to the gain coefficient g_l described in Chapter 2 as follows [see Eq. (1-3)]:

$$g_{tn} = g_t(\omega_n) = cg_l(\omega_n) \tag{3-7}$$

where c is the velocity of light.

The amplitude and frequency of oscillations in a gas laser are determined by two equations, which Lamb calls the "self-consistency" equations. The first of these equations states that the fractional rate of change of amplitude for an oscillation is equal to the gain coefficient for the oscillation minus the loss coefficient for the oscillation.[4] In the notation introduced above, we thus have

$$\frac{1}{E_n} \frac{dE_n}{dt} = \frac{1}{2}(g_{tn} - \alpha_{tn}) \tag{3-8}$$

The second self-consistency equation states that the frequency of an

---

[2] The assumption that the fields in the cavity are plane waves implies that E has only a z variation. E can be interpreted as one component (say, E_x) of a vector field in the xy plane.

[3] Usually, $\dot{\varphi}_n$ can be assumed to be zero, in which case the mode frequencies are given simply by the ω_n. In general, however, it is necessary to keep track of time-varying phase differences between different longitudinal modes. Thus $\varphi_n = \varphi_n(t)$, and $\dot{\varphi}_n$ appears formally as a frequency correction.

[4] When there is no risk of confusion, we shall use the general term "gain coefficient" to describe either g_t or g_l.

oscillation in a gas laser is determined by the resonance condition for the cavity. Thus,

$$\omega_n + \dot{\varphi}_n = \frac{\Omega_n}{n_n} \qquad (3\text{-}9)$$

where n_n is the refractive index of the gas at the frequency $\omega_n + \dot{\varphi}_n$. Note that the factor $\frac{1}{2}$ appears on the right-hand side of Eq. (3-8) because g_{tn} and α_{tn} refer to the fractional rate of change of *intensity* of the fields; the fractional rate of change of *amplitude* of the fields is given by $\frac{1}{2}g_{tn}$ or $\frac{1}{2}\alpha_{tn}$. Note also that the oscillation frequencies $\omega_n + \dot{\varphi}_n$ would be identical to the cavity frequencies Ω_n if the refractive index due to anomalous dispersion were included in the optical length of the cavity. It is conventional to retain the separate identity of the two frequencies and to refer to the difference between them as "frequency pulling."

3-3 GENERAL DISCUSSION OF GAS-LASER OSCILLATIONS

The self-consistency equations (3-8) and (3-9) are the fundamental equations governing the amplitudes and frequencies of the longitudinal modes in a gas laser. Most of the discussion in the remainder of this chapter is devoted to the problem of determining the gain coefficients g_{tn} and the refractive indices α_{tn} needed to solve the self-consistency equations. To get some feeling of the nature of the problem, it is worth considering the magnitudes of the pertinent parameters describing a typical gas laser.

Let us consider, for purposes of discussion, a helium-neon 6328-Å laser having a length $L = 1$ m. Such a laser might have a gain coefficient $g_{10} \approx 0.1/\text{m}$, corresponding to a temporal gain coefficient[5] $g_{t0} \approx 3 \times 10^7/\text{sec}$. The Doppler width of the 6328-Å transition is typically[6] $4\pi\sqrt{\ln 2}\,\Delta\omega_D \approx 1.7$ GHz, and we may assume that the homogeneous linewidth is $\gamma' \approx 100$ MHz. The frequency difference between adjacent longitudinal modes of the cavity (called the "free spectral range" of the cavity) is $(\Omega_{n+1} - \Omega_n)/2\pi = 150$ MHz. If we assume that the mirrors have reflectance $r = 0.99$, then the loss coefficient[7] is $\alpha_t = 3 \times 10^6/\text{sec}$.

---

[5] g_{t0} is defined by analogy to g_{10}; that is, g_{t0} is the gain per unit time for a mode at line center, in the limit that the homogeneous linewidth is zero, and saturation can be neglected.

[6] Note that numerical values of frequencies correspond to linear, not angular, frequencies.

[7] We assume that diffraction loss can be neglected.

An examination of the above numbers leads to some interesting general conclusions about oscillations in gas lasers. For example, note that there are several longitudinal modes having resonance frequencies within the Doppler width of the 6328-Å transition. Since an atom having a Doppler-shifted resonance frequency ω' can only interact with radiation whose frequency is in the range of approximately $\omega' \pm \gamma'$, it follows that atoms moving with different velocities contribute to different longitudinal modes, and in general there will be a "multimode" oscillation in the laser (that is, simultaneous oscillation in several longitudinal modes). However, since the homogeneous linewidth γ' is an appreciable fraction of the frequency separation between adjacent longitudinal modes, these modes may possibly "compete" with each other.

Note that the gain coefficient g_{t0} greatly exceeds the loss coefficient α_t. Since the rate of change of amplitude in a longitudinal mode is equal to the gain coefficient minus the loss coefficient, and since in a steady-state oscillation the amplitude of a longitudinal mode cannot increase monotonically, it follows [see Eq. (3-8)] that, when the laser is oscillating, the gain coefficient must saturate to a value $g_{tn} = \alpha_{tn}$. The gain coefficient g_{t0} thus gives little or no information concerning the amplitudes of the various longitudinal modes; it is the way in which g_{t0} *saturates* that determines the mode amplitudes.

The phenomenon of gain saturation was considered in Chapter 2; however, discussion there was limited to the case of a monochromatic traveling wave incident on a gas discharge. This limitation does not correspond to the actual physical situation in a gas laser. In the first place, the fields in multimode gas lasers are not monochromatic; they contain frequencies corresponding to the oscillation frequencies of all the longitudinal modes which happen to be excited in the laser. This fact causes considerable complication in the theoretical analysis. Since the fields in the laser are strong enough to cause appreciable saturation effects, the rate-equation approximation is not valid. That is, when the nonlinear response of the system is taken into account, "beating" effects occur between the various longitudinal mode frequencies which cause what Lamb calls "population pulsations." The population difference $\rho_{aa} - \rho_{bb}$ in Eq. (2-44) then becomes a function of time and cannot be taken outside the integral (as is required in the rate-equation approximation).

A further complication concerning saturation in a gas laser comes from the fact that gas atoms move through a standing-wave field. If only a single longitudinal mode is oscillating, so that the field in the cavity is monochromatic, an atom moving in the cavity will "see" a perturbation that appears to contain two frequencies.

Consider a standing-wave field in a cavity given by

$$E(z,t) = E_0 \sin Kz \cos \omega t \qquad (3\text{-}10)$$

An atom which is excited to state a at a time t_0 at a position z_0 with velocity v in the z direction will "see" a perturbation

$$V_{\text{int}} = -pE_0 \sin \{K[z_0 + v(t - t_0)]\} \cos \omega t \qquad (3\text{-}11)$$

This equation can be simplified by defining a phase angle

$$\vartheta = K(z_0 - vt_0) - \frac{\pi}{2} \qquad (3\text{-}12)$$

We then have

$$V_{\text{int}} = \frac{-pE_0}{2} \{\cos [(\omega - Kv)t - \vartheta] + \cos [(\omega + Kv)t + \vartheta]\} \qquad (3\text{-}13)$$

The perturbation thus contains two frequencies, $(\omega + Kv)$ and $(\omega - Kv)$. These frequencies can be visualized as Doppler-shifted frequencies seen by the atom as it moves through the forward and backward traveling waves comprising the standing wave in the cavity. As seen by a stationary observer, the frequency emitted or absorbed by the atom is always ω; there are no population pulsations in the laser, since the field is monochromatic.

Since there are no population pulsations in the laser, the factor $(\rho_{aa} - \rho_{bb})$ can be taken outside the integral in Eq. (2-36). Thus for the special case of a single-mode laser, we can derive rate equations[8] equivalent to Eqs. (2-43) and (2-44), but now the rate constant becomes

$$R = \frac{\mu^2 E_0^2}{4\hbar^2} \left[\frac{\gamma'}{(\omega - \omega')^2 + \gamma'^2} + \frac{\gamma'}{(\omega + \omega' - 2\omega_0)^2 + \gamma'^2} \right] \qquad (3\text{-}14)$$

where ω is the frequency of the standing-wave field, ω' is the Doppler-shifted

---

[8] Since the perturbation V_{int} seen by an atom is explicitly dependent upon the time t_0 (in the phase factor ϑ), we cannot a priori use the "complete" density matrix $\rho(t)$ to describe the behavior of the system; we must consider "elementary" density matrices $\rho(t, t_{0i})$ describing "classes" of atoms excited at different times t_{0i}. However, since there are no population pulsations, each of the elementary density matrices will obey rate equations. If we assume that the elementary density matrices $\rho(t, t_{0i})$ contribute to the complete density matrix $\rho(t)$ with completely random phase, then $\rho(t)$ itself obeys rate equations. Such a simplification is not possible when population pulsations must be considered.

atomic resonance frequency, ω_0 is the "center" frequency of the Doppler-broadened transition, and γ' is the homogeneous linewidth.

3-4 THRESHOLD CONDITIONS

In Chapter 2 expressions were derived for the gain coefficient (2-92) and refractive index (2-93) of a gas. At the threshold for oscillation in a laser, saturation effects can be neglected, in which case

$$g_t(\omega) = \frac{g_{t0}}{\sqrt{\pi}} Z_i(\xi + i\eta) \tag{3-15}$$

and

$$n(\omega) = 1 - \frac{g_{t0}}{2\sqrt{\pi}\,\omega} Z_r(\xi + i\eta) \tag{3-16}$$

where

$$g_{t0} = cg_{l0} = \frac{\sqrt{\pi}\,\omega_0\mu^2\mathscr{I}_0}{\epsilon_0\hbar\,\Delta\omega_D} \tag{3-17}$$

and Z_r and Z_i are the real and imaginary parts of the plasma dispersion function

$$Z(\xi + i\eta) = Z\left(\frac{\omega - \omega_0}{\Delta\omega_D} + i\frac{\gamma'}{\Delta\omega_D}\right) \tag{3-18}$$

These expressions can be inserted in the self-consistency equations (3-8) and (3-9) to yield the threshold conditions for gas laser oscillations. For a steady-state oscillation, $\dot{E}_n = 0$, in which case Eq. (3-8) becomes simply

$$\alpha_t = g_{tn} = g_t(\omega_n) \tag{3-19}$$

At line center, using Eq. (3-2), we find that

$$\frac{c}{L}(1 - r) = \frac{g_{t0}}{\sqrt{\pi}} Z_i\left(i\frac{\gamma'}{\Delta\omega_D}\right) \equiv g'_{to} \tag{3-20}$$

where g'_{to} is the measured unsaturated gain coefficient at line center. This equation has a very simple interpretation in the wave analysis. The maximum unsaturated gain per pass is given by

$$G'_0 = g'_{to}\frac{L}{c} \tag{3-21}$$

so that Eq. (3-20) can be written as

$$G'_0 = 1 - r \tag{3-22}$$

Thus, at threshold the unsaturated gain per pass equals the loss per pass.

Equation (3-20) can be used to determine the threshold length for a gas laser. We have

$$L_T = \frac{c(1 - r)}{g'_{to}} \tag{3-23}$$

The oscillation frequency of a laser at threshold is determined by Eq. (3-9). We may take $\dot{\varphi}_n = 0$ without loss of generality, in which case we find that

$$\omega_n = \Omega_n + \frac{g_{to}(\omega_n)}{2\sqrt{\pi}} Z_r(\xi + i\eta) \tag{3-24}$$

The oscillation frequencies are thus displaced from the passive cavity resonances. Since $Z_r(\xi + i\eta)$ is greater than zero for $\omega_n > \omega_0$ and less than zero for $\omega_n < \omega_0$ (see Figure 2-1), the oscillation frequencies are always "pulled" toward line center. The amount of frequency pulling can be conveniently expressed by using the threshold condition (3-20) in Eq. (3-24). For a pure inhomogeneous line, upon expanding the plasma dispersion function to first order in $\xi = (\omega - \omega_0)/\Delta\omega_D$, we find that

$$\frac{\omega_n - \Omega_n}{\omega_0 - \omega_n} \approx \frac{1}{\sqrt{\pi}} \frac{\alpha_t}{\Delta\omega_D} \tag{3-25}$$

To get an idea of the magnitude of the frequency pulling, note that, for the typical helium-neon laser described in the preceding section, $\alpha_t \approx 3 \times 10^6$ and $\Delta\omega_D \approx 10^9$. The frequency pulling is thus on the order of one or two parts per thousand.

The validity of relation (3-25) is restricted to the region near line center. In general, we have

$$\omega_n - \Omega_n = \frac{\alpha_t}{2} \frac{Z_r(\xi + i\eta)}{Z_i(\xi + i\eta)} \tag{3-26}$$

This equation indicates that the magnitude of the frequency pulling will be somewhat greater than that predicted by the approximation in (3-25).

Note that, although the refractive index for the transition is proportional to the gain coefficient, the amount of frequency pulling at threshold is independent of the gain coefficient. This results from the fact that as the gain coefficient increases, the threshold decreases.

3–5   SINGLE-MODE LASER

As mentioned in Section 3–3, if only a single longitudinal mode is excited in a laser, the rate-equation approximation can be used to account for saturation effects. Instead of the rate constant given by Eq. (2-53), there is a new rate constant which takes into account the two Doppler-shifted frequencies

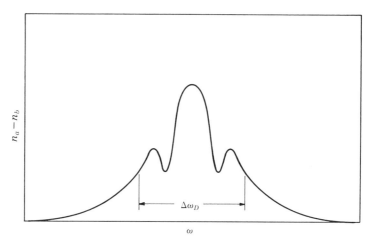

FIG. 3-1.   "Hole" burning in a standing-wave field.

seen by a moving atom [see Eq. (3-14)]. The saturated population difference $n_a - n_b$ [see Eq. (2-54)] is then given by

$$n_a - n_b = \frac{\mathscr{I}_0}{1 + \dfrac{\gamma \mu^2 E_0{}^2}{4\gamma' \gamma_a \gamma_b \hbar^2} \left[\dfrac{\gamma'}{(\omega - \omega')^2 + \gamma'^2} + \dfrac{\gamma'}{(\omega + \omega' - 2\omega_0)^2 + \gamma'^2} \right]}$$

(3-27)

In general (unless $\omega = \omega_0$), a standing wave burns *two* holes in the population difference $n_a - n_b$. This effect is to be contrasted with that caused by a traveling wave, which burns only one hole in the population difference $n_a - n_b$ (see Figure 2-2). The population difference as a function of Doppler-shifted frequency for the present situation is shown in Figure 3-1. Note that the two holes are symmetrically located with respect to line center.

The gain coefficient and refractive index for a single-mode laser can be derived by using procedures analogous to those of Chapter 2. The analysis proceeds in a straightforward manner until one arrives at the integral corresponding to Eq. (2-83), which again looks like

$$g_t(\omega) = \frac{g_{t0}\gamma'}{\pi} \int_0^\infty \frac{e^{-[(\omega' - \omega_0)/\Delta\omega_D]^2}}{(\omega - \omega')^2 + \gamma_s'^2} \, d\omega' \qquad (3\text{-}28)$$

where

$$g_{t0} = \frac{\sqrt{\pi} \, \omega_0 \mu^2 \mathscr{I}_0}{\epsilon_0 \hbar \, \Delta\omega_D} \qquad (3\text{-}29)$$

and

$$\gamma_s' = \gamma' \left(1 + \frac{W}{W_s}\right)^{1/2} \qquad (3\text{-}30)$$

but now there is a complication in that the saturation parameter is given by

$$W_s = 2W_{s0} \left[1 + \frac{2(\omega - \omega_0)(\omega' - \omega_0)}{(\omega - \omega_0)^2 + (\omega' - \omega_0)^2 + \gamma'^2}\right] \qquad (3\text{-}31)$$

The saturation parameter is thus a function of the integration variable ω', which of course means that γ_s' is a function of ω', and the integral in Eq. (3-28) cannot be evaluated in the simple form found in Chapter 2. It is possible, however, to eliminate the ω' dependence of the saturation parameter by making a fairly plausible approximation.

Note that at $\omega = \omega_0$ the saturation parameter is given by

$$W_s = 2W_{s0} \qquad (3\text{-}32)$$

that is, it is independent of ω'. In addition, if $\omega - \omega_0 \gg \gamma'$, that is, if the holes burned in the population difference versus frequency curve do not overlap, then we may take $\omega' - \omega_0 \approx \omega - \omega_0$, in which case the saturation parameter becomes

$$W_s = 4W_{s0} \qquad (3\text{-}33)$$

and again W_s is independent of ω'. In the region near line center, where the holes partially overlap, the population difference saturates over a frequency range of $\sim 2\gamma'$.

The above considerations lead us to assume that we can approximate the physical behavior[9] of the saturation parameter by replacing $(\omega' - \omega_0)$ by

[9] Note that this approximation becomes exact both for $\omega - \omega_0 \gg \gamma'$ and for $\omega = \omega_0$. Its major limitation is that it does not give the exact frequency dependence of W_s near line center, although it does indicate the approximate range of saturation.

$(\omega - \omega_0)$ in Eq. (3-31) and also replacing γ' by $2\gamma'$. With these approximations, and after some algebra, we find that Eq. (3-31) becomes

$$W_s = 4W_{s0}\left[\frac{1}{1 + \dfrac{\gamma'^2}{(\omega - \omega_0)^2 + \gamma'^2}}\right] \tag{3-34}$$

Having removed the ω' dependence in the saturation parameter, we can proceed to integrate Eq. (3-28). The result will, of course, be the same as that obtained in Chapter 2, namely, that [see Eq. (2-92)]

$$g_t(\omega) = \frac{g_{t0}}{\sqrt{\pi}\,[1 + (W/W_s)]^{\frac{1}{2}}}\, Z_i(\xi + i\eta) \tag{3-35}$$

By an analogous procedure, we find that the refractive index is given by [see Eq. (2-93)]

$$n(\omega) = 1 - \frac{g_{t0}}{2\sqrt{\pi}\,\omega}\, Z_r(\xi + i\eta) \tag{3-36}$$

where again Z_r and Z_i are the real and imaginary parts of the plasma dispersion function,

$$Z(\xi + i\eta) = Z\left[\frac{\omega - \omega_0}{\Delta\omega_D} + i\frac{\gamma'}{\Delta\omega_D}\left(1 + \frac{W}{W_s}\right)^{\frac{1}{2}}\right] \tag{3-37}$$

The gain coefficient (3-35) can now be inserted in the self-consistency equation (3-8) to determine the amplitude of oscillations in a single-frequency laser. For a steady-state oscillation, $\dot{E}_n = 0$, in which case Eq. (3-8) becomes

$$\alpha_t = \frac{g_{t0}}{\sqrt{\pi}\,[1 + (W/W_s)]^{\frac{1}{2}}}\, Z_i(\xi + i\eta) \tag{3-38}$$

This equation determines the intensity of oscillations in the laser. That is, the intensity W in the cavity will build up to a level such that the gain coefficient g_t saturates to a value equal to the loss coefficient α_t. The output intensity of the laser is then equal to this intensity times the transmittance of the laser mirrors.

The solution of Eq. (3-38) for the saturated "intracavity" intensity W is in general fairly complicated, since saturation effects occur not only in the denominator on the right-hand side, but also in the argument of the plasma dispersion function [see Eq. (3-37)].

Although detailed discussion of the output intensity of single-mode lasers will be delayed until Chapter 6, it is interesting to note at this time the general frequency dependence of the saturated intracavity intensity W. To this end, assume that the transition is pure inhomogeneous, so that $\gamma' \ll \Delta\omega_D$. Then,

$$Z_i(\xi + i\eta) \approx \sqrt{\pi}\, e^{-[(\omega - \omega_0)/\Delta\omega_D]^2} \tag{3-39}$$

Equation (3-38) can now be solved for the intracavity intensity. We find, after some algebra, that

$$W = W_s(X^2 e^{-2[(\omega - \omega_0)/\Delta\omega_D]^2} - 1) \tag{3-40}$$

where

$$X \equiv \frac{g_{t0}}{\alpha_t} = \frac{\sqrt{\pi}\, \omega_0 \mu^2 \mathcal{I}_0 L}{c(1 - r)\epsilon_0 \hbar\, \Delta\omega_D} \tag{3-41}$$

is called the "excitation parameter."[10] The excitation parameter can be described in terms of the threshold length of the laser:

$$X = \frac{L}{L_T} \tag{3-42}$$

Using Eq. (3-34), we can write (3-40) as

$$W = 4W_{s0} \left[\frac{X^2 e^{-2[(\omega - \omega_0)/\Delta\omega_D]^2} - 1}{1 + \dfrac{\gamma^2}{(\omega - \omega_0)^2 + \gamma'^2}} \right] \tag{3-43}$$

This equation indicates that there will be a "dip" in the intracavity intensity (and hence the output intensity) when the oscillation frequency of the laser is tuned to line center. The origin of this dip, called the "Lamb dip," can be understood by noting that when the laser is tuned to line center, only one hole is burned in the population difference versus frequency curve; whereas away from line center, two holes are burned in this curve. There are thus roughly twice as many atoms available to contribute to the laser oscillation when $\omega - \omega_0 > \gamma'$ as there are when $\omega = \omega_0$, so that the intracavity power shows a dip at line center, as shown in Figure 3-2.

The frequency of oscillation in a single-mode laser can be determined by using Eq. (3-36) for the refractive index in the self-consistency equation (3-9). Again, we can neglect $\dot{\varphi}_n$ without loss of generality. We obtain an equation

[10] Note that, for a pure inhomogeneous line, $g'_{to} = g_{to}$.

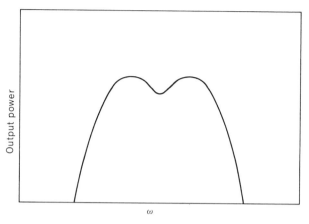

FIG. 3-2.   The "Lamb dip."

which looks identical to the threshold equation (3-24),

$$\omega_n = \Omega_n + \frac{g_{tn}}{2\sqrt{\pi}} Z_r(\xi + i\eta) \qquad (3\text{-}44)$$

but now the broadening parameter η depends on the intracavity intensity; that is,

$$\eta = \frac{\gamma'}{\Delta\omega_D}\left(1 + \frac{W}{W_s}\right)^{\frac{1}{2}} \qquad (3\text{-}45)$$

We see from Figure 2-1 that the amount of frequency pulling predicted by Eq. (3-44) becomes smaller as the broadening parameter η becomes larger. It thus follows that as the intracavity intensity increases, the magnitude of the frequency pulling will be reduced. This effect is sometimes called "frequency pushing." Note that, because of the frequency dependence of the saturation parameter, the frequency-pushing effect will be enhanced at line center.

3–6   MULTIMODE LASER

In a laser oscillating simultaneously in several longitudinal modes, a number of effects are observed which are not seen in single-mode lasers. In this section we shall describe these effects and determine their general origin. A "complete" treatment of saturation effects in a multimode laser has not yet been developed, and we shall restrict our attention to Lamb's "third-order" solution. Even with this limitation, the theory is fairly complicated; fortunately (perhaps), the complexity of the theory resides primarily in the mathematics, not in the physics. The essential features of multimode oscillations in gas lasers can be determined by considering a "three-mode" laser, and we shall restrict our attention to this case.

The field in a three-mode laser will comprise three monochromatic oscillations having frequencies at or near three cavity resonance frequencies. Assume that the oscillations correspond to adjacent cavity resonance frequencies, so that the frequency difference between them is given by

$$\Delta = \frac{\pi c}{L} \approx \omega_2 - \omega_1 \approx \omega_3 - \omega_2 \qquad (3\text{-}46)$$

As noted in Section 3-3, a typical value of $\Delta/2\pi$ might be 150 MHz.

We may begin our discussion by noting that a radiation field comprising three different monochromatic frequencies cannot have a constant intensity. Suppose that we have three oscillations

$$\begin{aligned}
A_1(t) &= \cos [\omega t + \varphi_1] \\
A_2(t) &= \cos [(\omega + \Delta)t + \varphi_2] \\
A_3(t) &= \cos [(\omega + 2\Delta)t + \varphi_3]
\end{aligned} \qquad (3\text{-}47)$$

The total field $A(t)$ is, of course,

$$A(t) = A_1(t) + A_2(t) + A_3(t) \qquad (3\text{-}48)$$

and the intensity[11] is

$$W(t) \propto \langle A^2(t) \rangle \qquad (3\text{-}49)$$

where the sign $\langle \ \rangle$ indicates a time average over a time long compared with $2\pi/\omega$, but short compared with times like $2\pi/\Delta$. Inserting Eqs. (3-47) and (3-48) in (3-49) and using standard trigonometric identities, we find that the intensity of the field is given by

$$W(t) \propto \frac{3}{2} + 2 \cos \left(\frac{2\varphi_2 - \varphi_1 - \varphi_3}{2} \right) \cos \Delta t + 2 \cos 2\Delta t \qquad (3\text{-}50)$$

This equation illustrates two fundamental characteristics of oscillations in multimode lasers. First, as noted above, the intensity is not constant but has components which fluctuate (in this case) at frequencies Δ and 2Δ. Second, the detailed behavior of $W(t)$ depends critically on the "relative phase factor" $2\varphi_2 - \varphi_1 - \varphi_3$. For example, if $2\varphi_2 - \varphi_1 - \varphi_3 = \pi$, then the fluctuation at Δ disappears altogether.

---

[11] This is sometimes called the "instantaneous intensity."

These observations lead to some interesting conclusions concerning the theoretical analysis of multimode lasers. Since the intensity of the field in the cavity fluctuates in time, the saturation of the gain coefficient must fluctuate in time. There will thus be "population pulsations" in the gas, as described in Section 3-3, and the rate-equation approximation cannot be used to describe the laser. In addition, since the intensity of the field depends on the relative phases of the different modes, it is important to keep track of the phase in the theoretical analysis.

Some insight into the general nature of the solution for the amplitudes and frequencies of oscillations in a three-mode laser can be gained by considering the third-order saturation behavior of a single-mode laser. For a single-mode laser, the gain coefficient saturates according to

$$g_t(\omega) = \frac{g_{t0}}{\sqrt{\pi}\,[1 + (W/W_s)]^{1/2}}\, Z_i(\xi + i\eta) \tag{3-51}$$

as described in the preceding section.

We assume in this section that the laser transition is pure inhomogeneous, so that Eq. (3-51) becomes

$$g_t(\omega) = \frac{g_{t0}e^{-\xi^2}}{[1 + (W/W_s)]^{1/2}} \tag{3-52}$$

We further assume that the laser is operating near threshold, so that $W \ll W_s$, in which case Eq. (3-52) can be expanded as

$$g_t(\omega) = g_{t0}e^{-\xi^2} - \frac{g_{t0}W}{2W_s} \tag{3-53}$$

where we neglect the frequency dependence in the saturation term. This equation can be inserted in the self-consistency equation (3-8) to yield

$$\dot{E}_1 = (\tfrac{1}{2}g_{t0}e^{-\xi^2} - \tfrac{1}{2}\alpha_t)E_1 - \frac{g_{t0}W}{4W_s}E_1 \tag{3-54}$$

Let

$$\alpha_1 \equiv \tfrac{1}{2}g_t e^{-\xi^2} - \tfrac{1}{2}\alpha_t \tag{3-55}$$

and

$$\beta_1 = \frac{c\epsilon_0}{8}\frac{g_{t0}}{W_s} = \frac{c\epsilon_0}{32}\frac{g_{t0}}{W_{s0}}\,[1 + \gamma^2\mathscr{L}(\omega - \omega_0)] \tag{3-56}$$

where [12]

$$\mathscr{L}(\omega - \omega_0) \equiv \frac{1}{(\omega - \omega_0)^2 + \gamma^2} \tag{3-57}$$

---

[12] In this section the effects of collision broadening are neglected.

Using these definitions, together with the relation $W = (c\epsilon_0/2)E_1{}^2$, we can write Eq. (3-54) as

$$\dot{E}_1 = \alpha_1 E_1 - \beta_1 E_1{}^3 \tag{3-58}$$

This last equation can be taken as the fundamental amplitude-determining equation in the "third-order" theory of a single-mode laser. We see that the growth in amplitude of the oscillation is limited by a saturation term $-\beta_1 E_1{}^3$. Note that the lowest-order saturation term is cubic; there are no terms proportional to $E_1{}^2$ which have the proper frequencies to "drive" the mode.

The same general saturation as that indicated by Eq. (3-58) occurs for a three-mode laser, except that the presence of three frequencies gives rise to several cubic terms which have the proper frequencies to drive the modes of the laser. Let the modes be denoted by

$$
\begin{aligned}
A_1(t) &= E_1 \cos (\omega_1 t + \varphi_1) \\
A_2(t) &= E_2 \cos (\omega_2 t + \varphi_2) \\
A_3(t) &= E_3 \cos (\omega_3 t + \varphi_3)
\end{aligned}
\tag{3-59}
$$

where E_1, E_2, E_3, φ_1, φ_2, and φ_3 are slowly varying functions of time. As noted before, we may assume that

$$\omega_2 - \omega_1 \approx \omega_3 - \omega_2 \approx \Delta = \frac{\pi c}{L} \tag{3-60}$$

but because of "frequency pulling" effects, we should expect that $\omega_2 - \omega_1$ might not be quite equal to $\omega_3 - \omega_2$.

To determine the saturation terms for a three-mode laser, note that

$$
\begin{aligned}
(A_1 + A_2 + A_3)^3 = {}&A_1{}^3 + A_2{}^3 + A_3{}^3 \\
&+ 3(A_1 A_2{}^2 + A_1 A_3{}^2 + A_2 A_1{}^2 + A_2 A_3{}^2 \\
&+ A_3 A_1{}^2 + A_3 A_2{}^2 + 2A_1 A_2 A_3)
\end{aligned}
\tag{3-61}
$$

This expression contains 27 terms having frequencies corresponding to the combinations of $(\cos \omega_1 t + \cos \omega_2 t + \cos \omega_3 t)^3$; however, most of these frequencies fall outside the linewidth of the laser transition and will not affect the saturation of the gain coefficients for the modes. The terms which have frequencies near a particular mode frequency and which, consequently, can "drive" the mode can be found by inspection from Eq. (3-61). Consider, for example, the terms having frequency components at ω_1. There are three such terms: $A_1{}^3$, $A_1 A_2{}^2$, and $A_1 A_3{}^2$. In addition, there is another term, $A_3 A_2{}^2$, which has a frequency component at $2\omega_2 - \omega_3$; since $\omega_2 - \omega_1 \approx$

$\omega_3 - \omega_2$, this frequency will also lie close to ω_1. In the present interpretation, these signals "beat" with the mode $A_1(t) = E_1 \cos(\omega_1 t + \varphi_1)$ to produce saturation terms which limit the amplitude of the mode. For the mode at ω_2, the appropriate terms are produced by A_2^3, $A_2 A_1^2$, $A_2 A_3^2$, and $A_1 A_2 A_3$; at ω_3, by A_3^3, $A_3 A_1^2$, $A_3 A_2^2$, and $A_1 A_2^2$.

We may thus conclude, reasoning by analogy to the amplitude-determining equation (3-58) for a single-mode laser, that the amplitude-determining equations for a three-mode laser should be of the form

$$\dot{E}_1 = \alpha_1 E_1 - \beta_1 E_1{}^3 - \vartheta_{12} E_1 E_2{}^2 - \vartheta_{13} E_1 E_3{}^2$$
$$- (\eta_{23} \cos \psi + \xi_{23} \sin \psi) E_2{}^2 E_3 \quad (3\text{-}62)$$

$$\dot{E}_2 = \alpha_2 E_2 - \beta_2 E_2{}^3 - \vartheta_{21} E_2 E_1{}^2 - \vartheta_{23} E_2 E_3{}^2$$
$$- (\eta_{13} \cos \psi + \xi_{13} \sin \psi) E_1 E_2 E_3 \quad (3\text{-}63)$$

$$\dot{E}_3 = \alpha_3 E_3 - \beta_3 E_3{}^3 - \vartheta_{31} E_3 E_1{}^2 - \vartheta_{32} E_3 E_2{}^2$$
$$- (\eta_{21} \cos \psi + \xi_{21} \sin \psi) E_2{}^2 E_1 \quad (3\text{-}64)$$

where ψ is the relative phase angle defined by

$$\psi = (2\omega_2 - \omega_1 - \omega_3)t + (2\varphi_2 - \varphi_1 - \varphi_3) \quad (3\text{-}65)$$

Using the same reasoning as that leading to Eqs. (3-62) through (3-64), we could write down by inspection the form of the frequency-determining equations that should be expected for a three-mode laser. We would find

$$\omega_1 + \dot{\varphi}_1 = \Omega_1 + \sigma_1 + \rho_1 E_1{}^2 + \tau_{12} E_2{}^2 + \tau_{13} E_3{}^2$$
$$+ (\eta_{23} \sin \psi - \xi_{23} \cos \psi) \frac{E_2{}^2 E_3}{E_1} \quad (3\text{-}66)$$

$$\omega_2 + \dot{\varphi}_2 = \Omega_2 + \sigma_2 + \rho_2 E_2{}^2 + \tau_{21} E_1{}^2 + \tau_{23} E_3{}^2$$
$$+ (\eta_{13} \sin \psi - \xi_{13} \cos \psi) E_1 E_3 \quad (3\text{-}67)$$

$$\omega_3 + \dot{\varphi}_3 = \Omega_3 + \sigma_3 + \rho_3 E_3{}^2 + \tau_{31} E_1{}^2 + \tau_{32} E_2{}^2$$
$$+ (\eta_{21} \sin \psi - \xi_{21} \cos \psi) \frac{E_2{}^2 E_1}{E_3} \quad (3\text{-}68)$$

The discussion given above might (charitably) be called heuristic, but when the third-order theory is carried out in detail, the amplitude and frequency-determining equations are precisely of the type given by Eqs. (3-62) to (3-64) and (3-66) to (3-68). The basic problem in the third-order theory is to determine the behavior of the coefficients in these equations.

Some insight into the physical significance of the coefficients in these equations can be gained by writing the amplitude equations in a somewhat different form. For example, let us rewrite Eq. (3-62) thus:

$$\frac{\dot{E}_1}{E_1} = \alpha_1 - \beta_1 E_1{}^2 - \vartheta_{12} E_2{}^2 - \vartheta_{13} E_3{}^2 - (\eta_{23} \cos \psi + \xi_{23} \sin \psi) \frac{E_2{}^2 E_3}{E_1}$$

$$(3\text{-}69)$$

By comparing this equation to Eq. (3-54), we conclude that α_1 gives the net unsaturated gain for the mode and that the other terms represent saturation effects. β_1 represents saturation of the mode by itself. (In fact, α_1 and β_1 turn out to have the same values in a three-mode laser as they do in a single-mode laser.)

The ϑ terms in Eq. (3-69) can be interpreted by using the concept of hole burning. For example, ϑ_{12} represents the saturation of mode 1 by the intensity in mode 2. This effect can be visualized as arising from the overlapping of holes burned in the population-difference versus frequency curve by the two modes. Note that, since each mode burns two holes symmetrically located with respect to line center, the "cross-saturation" effects represented by the ϑ's may be large even when the modes are not close together in frequency. The ξ and η terms are perhaps not so easy to visualize. These can be interpreted as saturation terms caused by intensity at or near one mode frequency which is created by "intermodulation distortion" between the other two modes. Lamb calls these terms "combination tones."

A similar physical interpretation can be given to the saturation coefficients in the frequency-determining equations, (3-66) through (3-68). Thus, the σ's represent the first-order frequency pulling; the ρ's represent frequency pushing of the type described for a single-mode laser; and the τ's represent pulling or pushing caused by cross-saturation effects. The ξ and η terms give rise to frequency modulation of a mode due to intermodulation distortion between the other modes.

We have not yet considered the problem of determining the magnitude of the various saturation coefficients. Unfortunately, this is not a problem which can be solved by using the qualitative arguments we have employed so far. As mentioned before, the basic difficulty in the theory of a multimode laser comes from the fact that the rate-equation approximation is not valid. This causes considerable complication in the theoretical analysis; and we shall only sketch Lamb's derivation of the saturation coefficients and quote the results here.

Since the rate-equation approximation is not valid, the behavior of the system cannot be described by a "complete" density matrix $\rho(t)$, which includes contributions from all atoms excited at times $t_0 < t$. Instead, we must consider each of the "classes" of atoms individually. By *classes* of atoms, we refer to all those atoms which would be included in a simple ensemble average over the atomic system. Thus, in the present situation we must use an "elementary" density matrix corresponding to all those atoms which are excited to state a at time t_0 at position $\vec{r_0}$ with velocity $\vec{v}$. To find the "complete" density matrix $\rho(\vec{r},t)$ for the system, we must add together all the elementary density matrices for atoms which are at some position $\vec{r}$ at some time t. Now the elementary density matrices $\rho(a,\vec{r_0},t_0,\vec{v},t)$ will obey equations of motion like (2-29), namely,

$$\dot{\rho}_{ab} = -(\gamma + i\omega_0)\rho_{ab} + iV(t)(\rho_{aa} - \rho_{bb}) \qquad (3\text{-}70)$$

$$\dot{\rho}_{aa} = -\gamma_a\rho_{aa} + iV(t)(\rho_{ab} - \rho_{ba}) \qquad (3\text{-}71)$$

$$\dot{\rho}_{bb} = -\gamma_b\rho_{bb} - iV(t)(\rho_{ab} - \rho_{ba}) \qquad (3\text{-}72)$$

$$\rho_{ba} = \rho_{ab}^* \qquad (3\text{-}73)$$

However, since $\rho_{aa} - \rho_{bb}$ is now a function of time, the off-diagonal elements cannot be "decoupled" from the on-diagonal elements, and we must deal with a set of coupled nonlinear equations. Lamb treats this problem with an iterative approach: He begins by assuming that, at t_0, $\rho_{aa} = 1$ and $\rho_{ab} = \rho_{ba} = \rho_{bb} = 0$. This initial condition yields a zero-order solution $\rho_{aa}^{(0)} = e^{-\gamma_a(t-t_0)}$, which is inserted in Eq. (3-70) to obtain a first-order solution $\rho_{ab}^{(1)}$. This solution is then used in Eqs. (3-71) and (3-72) to obtain improved solutions $\rho_{aa}^{(2)}$ and $\rho_{bb}^{(2)}$ for the diagonal elements of the elementary density matrix. The second-order solution is then reinserted in Eq. (3-70) to obtain the third-order solution $\rho_{ab}^{(3)}$.

The calculation is obviously very complicated. Not only does it involve a triple time integration, but once the behavior of an elementary density matrix has been determined, the contributions from all the elementary density matrices pertaining to atoms excited at a point $\vec{r_0}$ at time t_0 with velocity $\vec{v}$ such that they arrive at a point $\vec{r}$ at time t must be added together to obtain a complete density matrix $\rho(\vec{r},t)$ for the system. The whole procedure must then be repeated for atoms which were initially excited to state b. The polarization of the gas can then be determined by methods analogous to those employed in Chapter 2.

The final result of the calculation is to produce a set of equations like (3-62) to (3-64) and (3-66) to (3-68), which determine the amplitudes and frequencies of modes in a three-mode laser. We have tabulated Lamb's expressions[13] for the coefficients which enter these equations in Table 3-1.

Note that symbols such as ω_{12} appear in the table; these are simply abbreviations:

$$\omega_{12} \equiv \frac{\omega_1 + \omega_2}{2} \qquad (3\text{-}74)$$

In addition, note that the symbols $\mathscr{I}_2$ and $\mathscr{I}_4$ appear in the expressions for most of the saturation coefficients. These have a physical significance: they represent the effects of "spatial" competition between different modes. When several modes oscillate simultaneously in a laser, the competition between them will depend on the overlapping of their standing-wave patterns. For example, the standing-wave patterns of adjacent longitudinal modes are coincident near the mirrors of the laser, but in the center of the cavity the poles of the standing-wave pattern for one mode correspond to the zeros of the standing-wave pattern for the other mode.

Lamb accounts for these space-competition effects by defining "spatial Fourier components" of the inversion density

$$\mathscr{I}_{2(m-n)} = \frac{1}{L} \int_0^L \mathscr{I}_0(z,t) \cos 2(m-n)\frac{\pi z}{L}\, dz \qquad (3\text{-}75)$$

$\mathscr{I}_{2(m-n)}$ describes the space competition between the mth and nth longitudinal modes. Note that, if the inversion density is not a function of position, then all the spatial Fourier components vanish except $\mathscr{I}_0$. To simplify the discussion in this section, we shall assume that the inversion density is a constant function of position, so that terms involving $\mathscr{I}_2$ or $\mathscr{I}_4$ can be neglected. Thus we can neglect the ξ terms in Table 3-1.

Several interesting observations concerning the general operation of multimode lasers can now be made, using the amplitude and frequency equations (3-62) to (3-64) and (3-66) to (3-68), together with the values of the coefficients given in Table 3-1.

We may begin by noting the distinction between "weakly coupled" modes and "strongly coupled" modes. A mode is said to be weakly coupled if its saturation is primarily determined by a β coefficient; conversely, a mode is said to be strongly coupled if its saturation is primarily determined by a ϑ coefficient.

---

[13] Our notation is somewhat different from Lamb's.

TABLE 3–1 LAMB COEFFICIENTS

$$\alpha_n = \frac{g_{t0}}{2\sqrt{\pi}} Z_i \left(\frac{\omega_0 - \omega_n}{\Delta\omega_D} + i \frac{\gamma}{\Delta\omega_D} \right) - \frac{1}{2} \alpha_t$$

$$\beta_n = A[1 + \gamma^2 \mathscr{L}(\omega_0 - \omega_n)]$$

$$\vartheta_{12} = A\left\{ \gamma^2 \mathscr{L}(\omega_0 - \omega_{12}) + \frac{1}{\Delta^2} (\gamma_a{}^2 + \gamma_b{}^2) \right.$$

$$\left. + \frac{1}{\Delta^2} [\gamma^2 - (\omega_0 - \omega_1)\Delta] \frac{\mathscr{I}_2}{\mathscr{I}_0} \mathscr{L}(\omega_0 - \omega_1) \right\}$$

$$\vartheta_{21} = A\left\{ \gamma^2 \mathscr{L}(\omega_0 - \omega_{12}) + \frac{1}{\Delta^2} (\gamma_a{}^2 + \gamma_b{}^2) \right.$$

$$\left. + \frac{1}{\Delta^2} [\gamma^2 + (\omega_0 - \omega_2)\Delta] \frac{\mathscr{I}_2}{\mathscr{I}_0} \mathscr{L}(\omega_0 - \omega_2) \right\}$$

$$\vartheta_{13} = A\left\{ \gamma^2 \mathscr{L}(\omega_0 - \omega_{13}) + \frac{1}{4\Delta^2} (\gamma_a{}^2 + \gamma_b{}^2) \right.$$

$$\left. + \frac{1}{4\Delta^2} [\gamma^2 - 2(\omega_0 - \omega_1)\Delta] \frac{\mathscr{I}_4}{\mathscr{I}_0} \mathscr{L}(\omega_0 - \omega_1) \right\}$$

$$\vartheta_{31} = A\left\{ \gamma^2 \mathscr{L}(\omega_0 - \omega_{13}) + \frac{1}{4\Delta^2} (\gamma_a{}^2 + \gamma_b{}^2) \right.$$

$$\left. + \frac{1}{4\Delta^2} [\gamma^2 + 2(\omega_0 - \omega_3)\Delta] \frac{\mathscr{I}_4}{\mathscr{I}_0} \mathscr{L}(\omega_0 - \omega_3) \right\}$$

$$\vartheta_{23} = A\left\{ \gamma^2 \mathscr{L}(\omega_0 - \omega_{23}) + \frac{1}{\Delta^2} (\gamma_a{}^2 + \gamma_b{}^2) \right.$$

$$\left. + \frac{1}{\Delta^2} [\gamma^2 - (\omega_0 - \omega_2)\Delta] \frac{\mathscr{I}_2}{\mathscr{I}_0} \mathscr{L}(\omega_0 - \omega_2) \right\}$$

$$\vartheta_{32} = A\left\{ \gamma^2 \mathscr{L}(\omega_0 - \omega_{23}) + \frac{1}{\Delta^2} (\gamma_a{}^2 + \gamma_b{}^2) \right.$$

$$\left. + \frac{1}{\Delta^2} [\gamma^2 + (\omega_0 - \omega_3)\Delta] \frac{\mathscr{I}_2}{\mathscr{I}_0} \mathscr{L}(\omega_0 - \omega_3) \right\}$$

$$\eta_{23} = B\left\{ [\gamma^2 - (\omega_0 - \omega_{12})\Delta] \frac{\mathscr{I}_2}{\mathscr{I}_0} \mathscr{L}(\omega_0 - \omega_{12}) - 1 \right\}$$

$$\eta_{13} = B\left\{ [\gamma^2 + (\omega_0 - \omega_{23})\Delta] \frac{\mathscr{I}_2}{\mathscr{I}_0} \mathscr{L}(\omega_0 - \omega_{23}) \right.$$

$$\left. + [\gamma^2 - (\omega_0 - \omega_{12})\Delta] \frac{\mathscr{I}_2}{\mathscr{I}_0} \mathscr{L}(\omega_0 - \omega_{12}) + 2 \right\}$$

TABLE 3–1 LAMB COEFFICIENTS—*continued*

$$\eta_{21} = B\left\{[\gamma^2 - (\omega_0 - \omega_{23})\,\Delta]\,\frac{\mathscr{I}_2}{\mathscr{I}_0}\,\mathscr{L}(\omega_0 - \omega_{23}) - 1\right\}$$

$$\xi_{23} = C[(\omega_0 - \omega_{12} + \Delta)\mathscr{L}(\omega_0 - \omega_{12})]$$

$$\xi_{13} = C[(\omega_0 - \omega_{23} - \Delta)\mathscr{L}(\omega_0 - \omega_{23}) + (\omega_0 - \omega_{12} + \Delta)\mathscr{L}(\omega_0 - \omega_{12})]$$

$$\xi_{21} = C[(\omega_0 - \omega_{23} - \Delta)\mathscr{L}(\omega_0 - \omega_{23})]$$

$$\sigma_n = \frac{g_{t0}}{2\sqrt{\pi}}\,Z_r\!\left(\frac{\Omega_n - \omega_0}{\Delta\omega_D} + i\,\frac{\gamma}{\Delta\omega_D}\right)$$

$$\rho_n = D[(\omega_0 - \Omega_n)\mathscr{L}(\Omega_n - \omega_0)]$$

$$\tau_{12} = D\bigg[(\omega_0 - \omega_{12})\mathscr{L}(\omega_0 - \omega_{12}) + \frac{2}{\Delta}$$
$$+ \frac{\gamma_a\gamma_b}{\Delta^2}\,(\omega - \omega_1 + \Delta)\,\frac{\mathscr{I}_2}{\mathscr{I}_0}\,\mathscr{L}(\omega_0 - \omega_1)\bigg]$$

$$\tau_{21} = D\bigg[(\omega_0 - \omega_{12})\mathscr{L}(\omega_0 - \omega_{12}) - \frac{2}{\Delta}$$
$$+ \frac{\gamma_a\gamma_b}{\Delta^2}\,(\omega_0 - \omega_2 - \Delta)\,\frac{\mathscr{I}_2}{\mathscr{I}_0}\,\mathscr{L}(\omega_0 - \omega_2)\bigg]$$

$$\tau_{13} = D\bigg[(\omega_0 - \omega_{13})\mathscr{L}(\omega_0 - \omega_{13}) + \frac{1}{\Delta}$$
$$+ \frac{\gamma_a\gamma_b}{4\Delta^2}\,(\omega_0 - \omega_1 + 2\,\Delta)\,\frac{\mathscr{I}_2}{\mathscr{I}_0}\,\mathscr{L}(\omega_0 - \omega_1)\bigg]$$

$$\tau_{31} = D\bigg[(\omega_0 - \omega_{13})\mathscr{L}(\omega_0 - \omega_{13}) - \frac{1}{\Delta}$$
$$+ \frac{\gamma_a\gamma_b}{4\Delta^2}\,(\omega_0 - \omega_3 - 2\,\Delta)\,\frac{\mathscr{I}_2}{\mathscr{I}_0}\,\mathscr{L}(\omega_0 - \omega_3)\bigg]$$

$$\tau_{23} = D\bigg[(\omega_0 - \omega_{23})\mathscr{L}(\omega_0 - \omega_{23}) + \frac{2}{\Delta}$$
$$+ \frac{\gamma_a\gamma_b}{\Delta^2}\,(\omega_0 - \omega_2 + \Delta)\,\frac{\mathscr{I}_2}{\mathscr{I}_0}\,\mathscr{L}(\omega_0 - \omega_2)\bigg]$$

$$\tau_{32} = D\bigg[(\omega_0 - \omega_{23})\mathscr{L}(\omega_0 - \omega_{23}) - \frac{2}{\Delta}$$
$$+ \frac{\gamma_a\gamma_b}{\Delta^2}\,(\omega_0 - \omega_3 - \Delta)\,\frac{\mathscr{I}_2}{\mathscr{I}_0}\,\mathscr{L}(\omega_0 - \omega_3)\bigg]$$

$$A = \frac{c\epsilon_0}{32}\,\frac{g_{t0}}{W_{s0}} \qquad B = \frac{\gamma_a\gamma_b}{\Delta^2}\,A \qquad C = \gamma B\mathscr{I}_2 \qquad D = -\gamma A$$

Modes which are weakly coupled behave quite differently from modes which are strongly coupled. If a laser has only weakly coupled modes,[14] so that the β coefficients determine the saturation behavior, then to a first approximation Eqs. (3-62) to (3-64) reduce to a set of equations like (3-58), and the multimode laser behaves as an assemblage of independent single-mode lasers. On the other hand, if the modes are strongly coupled, the situation is quite different. The intensity in one mode will reduce the intensity in the mode to which it is coupled. In the extreme case, oscillation on one mode may prevent another mode from reaching threshold. (This is called "mode quenching.")

An examination of the ϑ coefficients in Table 3-1 shows that strong coupling occurs under two different conditions.[15] The first condition obtains when two modes are symmetrically located with respect to line center. In this case the factor $\gamma^2 \mathscr{L}(\omega_0 - \omega_{mn})$ has a maximum.[16] The other condition obtains when the cavity is long enough so that the frequency separation between adjacent longitudinal modes is comparable with the decay rates γ_a and γ_b.

The two conditions for strong coupling give rise to markedly different behavior of the modes. If the strong coupling is determined by the $\gamma^2 \mathscr{L}(\omega_0 - \omega_{mn})$ terms, the mode competition effects which occur are stationary in time. On the other hand, if the strong coupling is determined by the $(\gamma_a^2 + \gamma_b^2)/\Delta^2$ terms, then examination of Table 3-1 shows that the η terms are also important, in which case the saturation effects are, in general, functions of time, through the relative phase factor ψ.[17] Thus, when the η terms become important, the mode amplitudes become functions of time.

When the mode amplitudes are functions of time, the cross-saturation effects caused by the ϑ's will also be functions of time. Since the ϑ terms are larger than the η terms, they will tend to "amplify" the time-varying saturation effects caused by the η terms. In addition, since the oscillation frequencies which determine ψ are themselves functions of both the η terms and the cross-saturation terms τ_{mn}, one should expect ψ to vary as a complicated function of time. We thus conclude from these general considerations that the amplitudes and frequencies of modes in a long laser will normally have a complicated time dependence.

---

[14] Note that in general some of the modes of a multimode laser will be weakly coupled, whereas others will be strongly coupled.

[15] We neglect terms involving $\mathscr{I}_2$ or $\mathscr{I}_4$.

[16] This condition corresponds to the situation where the "second hole" burned by one mode overlaps the "first hole" burned by the other mode.

[17] To get a rough estimate of the general time variation of the relative phase factor ψ, note that pulling effects are typically measured in parts per thousand, so that we should expect ψ to vary at audio (as opposed to radio) frequencies.

The above considerations indicate that the "mode dynamics" in a three-mode laser are controlled by the relative phase factor ψ. It is therefore interesting to examine the time variation of ψ in greater detail. By subtracting Eqs. (3-66) and (3-68) from twice (3-67), we find a differential equation for ψ:[18]

$$\dot{\psi} = \sigma + A \sin \psi \qquad (3\text{-}76)$$

where

$$\sigma = 2\sigma_2 - \sigma_1 - \sigma_3 \qquad (3\text{-}77)$$

and

$$A = \frac{c\epsilon_0}{32} \frac{g_{t0}}{W_{s0}} \frac{\gamma_a \gamma_b}{\Delta^2} \left(\frac{4E_1{}^2 E_3{}^2 + E_1{}^2 E_2{}^2 + E_2{}^2 E_3{}^2}{E_1 E_3} \right) \qquad (3\text{-}78)$$

The solution of Eq. (3-76) for ψ depends critically on whether A is greater or less than σ. If $A < \sigma$, then there is no particular constraint on the solution $\psi = \psi(t)$. On the other hand, if $A > \sigma$, the only solution for Eq. (3-76) is $\psi = $ constant. This can be seen by noting that if $\dot{\psi}$ were zero, then A would not be a function of time [see Eqs. (3-62) to (3-64)]. Since σ is not a function of time, if $\dot{\psi} = 0$, then

$$\ddot{\psi} = \dot{\psi} A \cos \psi = 0 \qquad (3\text{-}79)$$

We conclude that if $\dot{\psi}$ ever becomes zero, then it will always remain zero. If $A > \sigma$, then $\dot{\psi}$ will become equal to zero[19] for

$$\psi = -\sin^{-1} \frac{\sigma}{A} \qquad (3\text{-}80)$$

and thereafter will always remain zero. ψ itself is then forced to remain constant in time, which in turn forces $\omega_2 - \omega_1 = \omega_3 - \omega_2$. When this condition obtains, the laser is said to be "phase-locked."

The condition for phase locking in a three-mode laser is that the modes be about symmetrically located with respect to line center. In this case, $\sigma_2 \approx 0$ and $\sigma_1 \approx -\sigma_3$, so that $\sigma \approx 0$.

The mode dynamics of a three-mode laser are markedly different if the modes are phase-locked rather than "free-running." If the modes are phase-locked, then none of the saturation terms in Eqs. (3-62) to (3-64) and (3-66) to (3-68) are functions of time, so that the amplitudes and frequencies of

---

[18] We neglect here the "frequency pushing" terms ρ_m and the "cross-saturation" terms τ_{mn}. It is also assumed that terms involving $\mathscr{I}_2$ and $\mathscr{I}_4$ can be neglected.

[19] A more rigorous analysis shows that ψ approaches zero asymptotically.

the modes will be constant in time. On the other hand, if the modes are free-running, there will always be time-varying saturation effects, so that there will always be some degree of amplitude and frequency modulation of the modes. As mentioned above, these modulation effects will become more prominent as the laser is made longer.

We may close by noting that all the theoretical predictions described in this chapter have been confirmed experimentally, so that Lamb's third-order theory of a three-mode laser can be considered to give at least a qualitative understanding of the physical processes occurring in multimode lasers. The basic problem with the third-order theory is, of course, that it is valid only at the onset of saturation phenomena. Thus we cannot expect to use the third-order theory to predict the output power of a laser, for example.

REFERENCES

1. W. E. Lamb, Jr., *Phys. Rev.*, **134**: A1429 (1964); W. E. Lamb, Jr., in P. A. Miles (ed.), "Quantum Electronics and Coherent Light," p. 78, Academic Press, Inc., New York, 1964.

The *Physical Review* paper is the classic paper in the field of gas lasers. The discussion in "Quantum Electronics and Coherent Light" is more tutorial, but unfortunately it contains numerous typographical errors.

2. R. L. Fork and M. A. Pollack, *Phys. Rev.*, **139**: A1408 (1965).

This paper extends Lamb's work to account for the effects of collisions. The discussion is limited to a two-mode laser and is not completely general.

4 TRANSVERSE MODE STRUCTURE

The fundamental reason for the importance of gas lasers as light sources is that the light emitted by them is confined to one, or at most to a few, radiation modes.

The general concept of modes in the optical region of the spectrum has been known for many years; the derivation of Planck's blackbody-radiation law, for example, utilizes the fact that in a closed optical cavity of unit volume there are $(8\pi\nu^2/c^3)\,d\nu$ modes having frequencies between ν and $(\nu + d\nu)$. The detailed characteristics of these modes are of little interest, since the amount of power radiated by an ordinary light source into any single mode is very small. Thus, before the advent of lasers the investigation of mode structure in various optical cavities was of no practical importance, and the only cavities for which the modes were known were ones where the characteristics of the modes could be determined by simple symmetry considerations. For example, in a cubical box having conducting walls, the modes must take the form of uniform-amplitude plane waves.

In a laser cavity such simple arguments are not sufficient to determine the characteristics of the modes. A laser cavity is an "open" cavity having no side walls, and its modes must be determined by considering the manner in which light propagates back and forth between the cavity mirrors.

The theory of laser mode structure has been developed by several workers, using a variety of different techniques. In this chapter we shall consider the numerical techniques introduced by Fox and Li to determine the modes of a plane-parallel cavity; the analytic solution for the modes of a confocal cavity developed by Boyd and Gordon; and the geometrical formalism introduced by Deschamps, Mast, and Laures for determining the characteristics of modes of general curved-mirror optical cavities.

As mentioned in Chapter 3, it is convenient to consider two different types of modes. A "transverse" mode of a cavity is a field distribution which repeats itself (to within a constant) upon making a complete traversal of the cavity. Corresponding to each transverse mode of a cavity are several "longitudinal" modes. A longitudinal mode is defined by the requirement that its frequency correspond to a cavity resonance. Thus the frequency of the mth longitudinal mode in a gas laser is given by [see Eq. (3-9)]

$$\omega_m + \dot{\varphi}_m = m \frac{\pi c}{n_m L} \qquad (4\text{-}1)$$

In this chapter we shall confine our attention to an investigation of mode structure in "passive" cavities (that is, cavities containing no amplifying media). The reason for this is that the transverse modes of a gas laser are approximately the same as the transverse modes of a passive cavity: the simplification of the analysis achieved by not considering the presence of an active medium in the cavity does not detract from the usefulness of the solution.

The longitudinal modes of an "active" cavity have been considered in detail in Chapter 3. The longitudinal modes of a passive cavity are comparatively uninteresting; they simply correspond to a "comb" of frequencies given by [see Eq. (3-1)]

$$\Omega_m = m \frac{\pi c}{L} \qquad (4\text{-}2)$$

Consequently, in this chapter the discussion will principally concern transverse mode structure, and the term "mode" will be used freely to mean "transverse mode."

4–1 PLANE-PARALLEL CAVITY

The optical cavity used in the first gas laser was the plane-parallel cavity, which consists of two plane mirrors separated by a distance L, as shown in Figure 4-1. The plane-parallel cavity has been studied in considerable detail by Fox and Li. In this section, we shall outline the method of their analysis and consider some of their results.

The modes of an optical cavity can be determined by a self-consistent field analysis: a field distribution on one of the mirrors which reproduces itself after a complete traversal of the cavity constitutes a mode of the cavity. Because of diffraction, only the *distribution* of field can be expected to reproduce itself; there will always be some loss of light around the edges of the

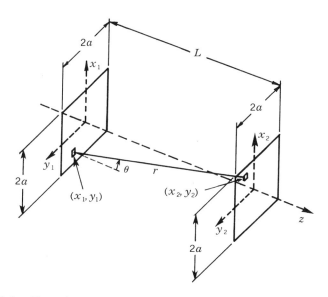

FIG. 4-1.   Illustration of the definition of variables in a plane-parallel cavity.

mirrors, and the absolute *magnitude* of the field must decrease after traversing the cavity. In addition, there will be a phase shift of $4\pi/\lambda$, where λ is the wavelength of the mode, which is accumulated by the field distribution in making a complete traversal of the cavity. The requirement that the phase of the field distribution return to its initial value (times some integer times 2π) determines the resonant wavelengths of the cavity. The longitudinal mode frequencies are then found from

$$\Omega_m = \frac{2\pi c}{\lambda_m} \qquad (4\text{-}3)$$

where c is the phase velocity of the mode.

In a plane-parallel cavity comprising two mirrors of identical size, a mode must have the same field distribution on each mirror. Thus it is sufficient in this case to consider a "single pass" rather than a complete traversal of the field distribution in a mode.

The effects of diffraction loss and phase shift are accounted for by a complex constant γ, which is called the "eigenvalue" for the mode. The real and imaginary parts of γ determine the loss and phase shift of a mode as it makes a single-pass traversal of the cavity.

The propagation of a field back and forth between the mirrors of an optical cavity can be determined by repeated applications of Huygens' principle.

Thus, if the field on one of the mirrors is given by $u_1(x_1, y_1)$, it will become $u_2(x_2, y_2)$ on the other mirror, where $u_2(x_2, y_2)$ is related to $u_1(x_1, y_1)$ by the Fresnel-Kirchhoff integral theorem:

$$u_2(x_2, y_2) = \frac{ik}{4\pi} \int \int_{S_1} u_1(x_1, y_1) \frac{e^{-ikr}}{r} (1 + \cos \vartheta) \, dx_1 \, dy_1 \qquad (4\text{-}4)$$

The integration range S_1 denotes an integration over the total area of mirror 1; r is the distance between the point (x_1, y_1) and the point (x_2, y_2); $k = 2\pi/\lambda$ is the wavenumber of the field; and $(1 + \cos \vartheta)$ is the so-called "obliquity factor," with ϑ being the angle between the axis of the system and the direction of r.

Consider a plane-parallel cavity comprising two square mirrors separated by a distance L, as shown in Figure 4-1. Let the field on one mirror be given by $u_1(x_1)v_1(y_1)$, and let the field on the other mirror be given by $u_2(x_2)v_2(y_2)$. Using Eq. (4-4), we then have

$$u_2(x_2)v_2(y_2) = \frac{ik}{4\pi} \int_{-a}^{a} \int_{-a}^{a} u_1(x_1)v_1(y_1) \frac{e^{-ikr}}{r} \left(1 + \frac{L}{r}\right) dx_1 \, dy_1 \quad (4\text{-}5)$$

where

$$r = \sqrt{L^2 + (x_2 - x_1)^2 + (y_2 - y_1)^2} \qquad (4\text{-}6)$$

If $L \gg a$, Eq. (4-5) can be simplified to

$$u_2(x_2)v_2(y_2) = \frac{ike^{-ikL}}{2\pi L} \int_{-a}^{a} \int_{-a}^{a} u_1(x_1)v_1(y_1)e^{-(ik/2L)[(x_2-x_1)^2+(y_2-y_1)^2]} \, dx_1 \, dy_1$$

$$(4\text{-}7)$$

According to the discussion above, we can determine the modes of a plane-parallel cavity by finding the field $u_2(x_2)v_2(y_2)$ caused by $u_1(x_1)v_1(y_1)$ using Eq. (4-7) and demanding that $u_2(x_2)v_2(y_2)$ and $u_1(x_1)v_1(y_1)$ be equal to within a complex constant. We thus obtain, noting that Eq. (4-7) is separable in x and y, two equations which determine the modes of a plane-parallel cavity:

$$u_m(x_2) = \gamma_m \frac{e^{i\pi/4}}{\sqrt{2\pi L/k}} \int_{-a}^{a} u_m(x_1)e^{-i(k/2L)(x_2-x_1)^2} \, dx_1 \qquad (4\text{-}8)$$

$$v_n(y_2) = \gamma_n \frac{e^{i\pi/4}}{\sqrt{2\pi L/k}} \int_{-a}^{a} v_n(y_1)e^{-i(k/2L)(y_2-y_1)^2} \, dy_1 \qquad (4\text{-}9)$$

where the phase shift e^{-ikL} has been incorporated in the γ's. The product $\gamma_m \gamma_n$ then gives the loss and phase shift *per pass*. We have written the field distributions in Eqs. (4-8) and (4-9) with subscripts m and n to allow for the possibility that there may be several different solutions of these equations.

Equations (4-8) and (4-9) are integral eigenvalue equations; the problem of determining the modes of a plane-parallel cavity is thus equivalent to the mathematical problem of determining the eigenfunctions of these equations.

The transverse modes of a cavity are conventionally designated by the notation "TEM_{mn}," where the field in the TEM_{mn} mode has the distribution $u_m(x)v_n(y)$. The modes are ordered according to the magnitude of the eigenvalues γ_m and γ_n, with the largest of the eigenvalues being assigned the lowest numbers. Thus the "lowest-loss" mode is the TEM_{00} mode, the next lowest is the TEM_{01} or TEM_{10} mode, and so forth.

Equations (4-8) and (4-9), which determine the modes of a plane-parallel cavity, involve Fresnel integrals that cannot be evaluated analytically. Fox and Li have used numerical integration techniques to solve these equations. Their general approach is to assume an initial field distribution on one mirror and allow the field to "propagate" back and forth between the mirrors, using Eqs. (4-8) and (4-9). After several passes they observe that the field $u(x)v(y)$ assumes a distribution which does not change from pass to pass. Such a field distribution is defined as a transverse mode of the cavity.

The critical parameter determining the general nature of the solutions of Eqs. (4-8) and (4-9) is the "Fresnel number" N, which is defined by

$$N = \frac{a^2}{L\lambda} \tag{4-10}$$

The Fresnel number determines the total number of oscillations of the exponential factors inside the integrals of Eqs. (4-8) and (4-9) over the integration range of x_1 and y_1.

Equations (4-8) and (4-9) are, of course, completely identical except for the interchange of x and y. Thus, in finding their solution, it suffices to consider only one of them. This corresponds to the problem of determining the modes of a cavity comprising "infinite-strip" mirrors.

Fox and Li's results for the two lowest-order modes of an infinite-strip plane-parallel cavity are shown in Figures 4-2 and 4-3. The lowest-order mode is seen to be an almost-plane wave whose amplitude is peaked at the center of the mirror and falls off toward the edge. The next-lowest-order mode has zero amplitude in the center of the mirror but still has an almost-plane wavefront. Note that the number of "ripples" in the amplitude and phase distributions depends on the Fresnel number N.

The general iterative technique described above can be used to study the modes of any optical cavity. Fox and Li have used the technique to study cavities comprising circular plane mirrors and confocal spherical mirrors.[1] For a cavity comprising circular plane mirrors, the modes are generally similar to the modes of a cavity comprising infinite-strip plane mirrors, except that the modes are azimuthally symmetric. For a confocal cavity, the modes are somewhat different. In particular, the amplitude and phase distributions in the modes of a confocal cavity do not contain the ripples

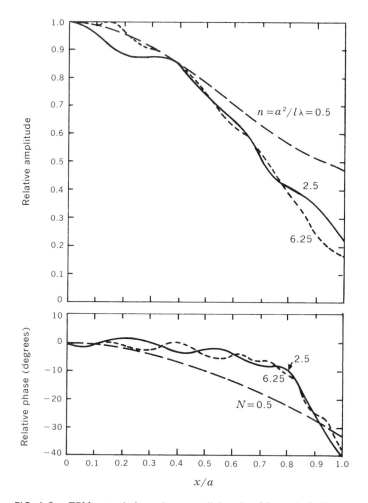

FIG. 4-2.   TEM$_{00}$ mode in a plane-parallel cavity. [*From A. G. Fox and T. Li, Bell Syst. Tech. J.*, **40**:453 (1961).]

---

[1] The confocal cavity comprises two spherical mirrors of equal radius of curvature, separated by a distance equal to their radius of curvature.

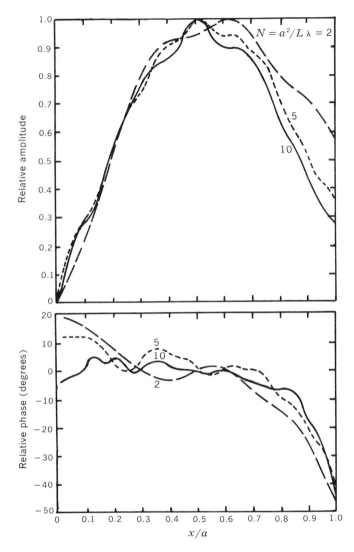

FIG. 4-3.   TEM$_{01}$ mode in a plane-parallel cavity. [*From A. G. Fox and T. Li, Bell Syst. Tech. J.,* **40**:453 (1961).]

found in the modes of a plane-parallel cavity. In addition, the modes of a confocal cavity are more concentrated along the axis of the cavity than are the modes of a plane-parallel cavity. The modes of a confocal cavity can be found by an analytic method, which will be described in the next section.

It is interesting to compare the eigenvalues obtained for the modes of a confocal cavity with those obtained for the modes of a plane-parallel cavity. Figure 4-4 shows the power losses per pass (determined by the magnitudes of the eigenvalues) for some low-order modes in plane-parallel and confocal cavities. We see that the diffraction losses for the modes of a confocal cavity are much less than for the modes of a plane-parallel cavity. In addition, the difference in the losses for adjacent-order modes is greater for a confocal

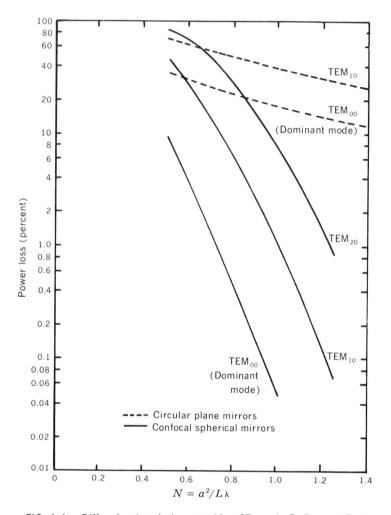

FIG. 4-4.   Diffraction loss in laser cavities. [*From A. G. Fox and T. Li, Bell Syst. Tech. J.*, **40**:453 (1961).]

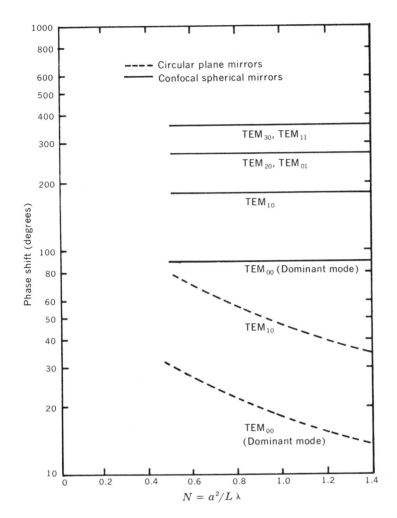

FIG. 4-5.   Phase shifts in laser cavities. [*From A. G. Fox and T. Li, Bell Syst. Tech. J.*, **40**:453 (1961).]

cavity than it is for a plane-parallel cavity. Thus a confocal cavity has better "mode discrimination" than does a plane-parallel cavity.

The single-pass phase shifts (determined by the arguments of the eigenvalues) for some low-order modes in confocal and plane-parallel cavities are shown in Figure 4-5. We see that the phase shift associated with a mode of a confocal cavity is independent of the Fresnel number, but that the phase shift associated with a mode of a plane-parallel cavity increases as the Fresnel number is reduced. The resonance frequencies of the modes in a plane-parallel cavity thus depend on the size of the mirrors.

The effects of nonparallelism between the mirrors of a nominally plane-parallel cavity have been studied by Fox and Li. Figure 4-6 shows the power

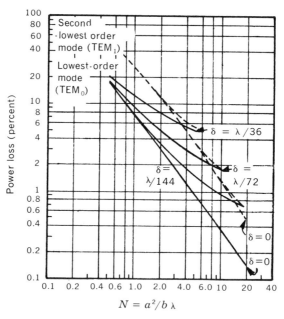

$$N = a^2/b\,\lambda$$

FIG. 4-6.   Diffraction loss for a misaligned plane-parallel cavity. [*From A. G. Fox and T. Li, Proc. IEEE*, **51**:80 (1963).]

loss per pass for the two lowest-order modes of an infinite-strip (nominally) plane-parallel cavity for various mirror tilts. The amplitude and phase distribution in the fundamental mode is shown in Figure 4-7. It is seen that, as the mirrors are tilted, the mode becomes asymmetric.

The plane-parallel cavity is not usually employed in practical laser systems. The reason for this can be seen from the curves shown in Figure 4-6. Using the data in this figure, one can calculate that in order to maintain the diffraction loss in a typical laser cavity (1 m long by 3 mm in diameter) below 1 percent per pass, it is necessary to maintain the parallelism of the mirrors to within 1 sec of arc. This is an extremely stringent requirement for a mechanical structure of this size. Fortunately, the alignment tolerance of curved-mirror cavities is much greater; most practical lasers employ curved-mirror cavities.

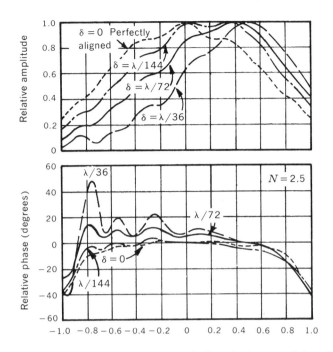

FIG. 4-7. Fundamental mode in a misaligned plane-parallel cavity. [*From A. G. Fox and T. Li, Proc. IEEE*, **51**:80 (1963).]

4–2 CONFOCAL CAVITY

As mentioned in the previous section, the modes of a confocal cavity are different from those of a plane-parallel cavity. Boyd and Gordon have shown that the modes of a confocal cavity can be determined by using analytical methods and can be approximated by functions which enable one to find the field distribution in any plane normal to the axis of the cavity, not just on the cavity mirrors. In this section, we shall outline the Boyd and Gordon solution and consider some of its implications.

A confocal cavity consists of two mirrors of equal radius of curvature b, separated by a distance equal to their radius of curvature, as shown in Figure 4-8. We shall assume in this section that the mirrors have a square cross-section of width $2a$.

The equations determining the modes of a confocal cavity are similar to (4-8) and (4-9), except that for a confocal cavity one can neglect the terms $x_2^2 - x_1^2$ and $y_2^2 - y_1^2$ in the exponentials on the right-hand side, so that

$$u_m(x_2) = \gamma_m \frac{e^{i\pi/4}}{\sqrt{2\pi b/k}} \int_{-a}^{a} u_m(x_1) e^{-i(k/b)(x_2 x_1)} \, dx_1 \qquad (4\text{-}11)$$

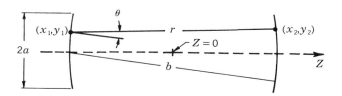

FIG. 4-8.   Illustration of the definition of variables for a confocal cavity.

and

$$v_n(y_2) = \gamma_n \frac{e^{i\pi/4}}{\sqrt{2\pi b/k}} \int_{-a}^{a} v_n(y_1) e^{-i(k/b)(y_2 y_1)} \, dy_1 \qquad (4\text{-}12)$$

The simplification achieved by the elimination of $x_2^2 - x_1^2$ and $y_2^2 - y_1^2$ from the equations defining the modes is significant; it reduces a problem in Fresnel diffraction to one in Fraunhofer diffraction. Boyd and Gordon have shown that the Fraunhofer-diffraction problem defined by Eqs. (4-11) and (4-12) has an analytic solution. In particular, they have shown that the eigenfunctions satisfying these equations are the angular wave functions in prolate-spheroidal coordinates:

$$u_m\left(c, \frac{x}{a}\right) v_n\left(c, \frac{y}{a}\right) = S_{0m}\left(c, \frac{x}{a}\right) S_{0n}\left(c, \frac{y}{a}\right) \qquad (4\text{-}13)$$

where

$$c = 2\pi N = 2\pi \frac{a^2}{b\lambda} \qquad (4\text{-}14)$$

In addition, they have shown that the eigenvalues of Eqs. (4-11) and (4-12) are given by[2]

$$\frac{1}{\gamma_{mn}} \equiv \frac{1}{\gamma_m \gamma_n} = 4Ni^{(1+m+n)} R_{0m}^{(1)}(c,1) R_{0n}^{(1)}(c,1) \qquad (4\text{-}15)$$

where $R_{0m}^{(1)}(c,1)$ and $R_{0n}^{(1)}(c,1)$ are the radial wave functions of the first kind in prolate-spheroidal coordinates.

The prolate-spheroidal wave functions are real; it therefore follows that the field distribution $u_m(c,x/a)v_n(c,y/a)$ of the TEM$_{mn}$ transverse mode has a constant phase across the cavity mirrors; that is, the wavefronts of the modes of a confocal cavity are spherical.

---

[2] The geometrical phase-shift factor e^{-ikb} has been omitted.

The total phase shift accumulated by the TEM_{mn} mode in a complete traversal of the cavity is given by

$$\varphi = 2\left[(1 + m + n)\frac{\pi}{2} - kb\right] \tag{4-16}$$

Since for resonance this must be equal to some integer q times 2π, we obtain the resonance condition for the confocal cavity, after some algebra:

$$\Omega = \frac{\pi c}{2b}(2q + 1 + m + n) \tag{4-17}$$

The integer q is the longitudinal mode number; for each transverse mode TEM_{mn} there are a series of longitudinal modes corresponding to different values of q. Note that the modes of a confocal cavity are highly degenerate: the qth longitudinal mode associated with the TEM_{mn} transverse mode has the same resonance frequency as the $(q - 1)$th longitudinal mode associated with the $\mathrm{TEM}_{m(n+2)}$ transverse mode, and so on. We see from Eq. (4-17) that the transverse modes of a confocal cavity can be grouped into two classes: "even-symmetric" modes, corresponding to $(m + n)$ being even, and "odd-symmetric" modes, corresponding to $(m + n)$ being odd. The longitudinal modes associated with each class are completely degenerate, and the longitudinal mode resonances corresponding to the even-symmetric transverse modes lie halfway between those corresponding to the odd-symmetric transverse modes.

The field distributions in the transverse modes of a confocal cavity can be determined from tabulated values of the angular-spheroidal wave functions, but much greater insight into the nature of the modes can be gained by using an approximation introduced by Boyd and Gordon. They have pointed out that, if the Fresnel number of the cavity is large compared with unity (a typical situation), the angular-spheroidal wave functions can be approximated with negligible error by Hermite-gaussian functions. In particular, the field distributions on the mirrors of a confocal cavity can be expressed as

$$u_m(x) = H_m\left(\frac{\sqrt{2}}{w_s}x\right)e^{-x^2/w_s{}^2} \tag{4-18}$$

and

$$v_n(y) = H_n\left(\frac{\sqrt{2}}{w_s}y\right)e^{-y^2/w_s{}^2} \tag{4-19}$$

TEM$_{00}$

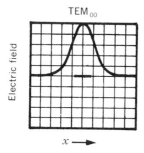

TEM$_{01}$

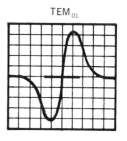

TEM$_{02}$

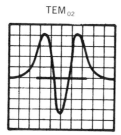

TEM$_{03}$

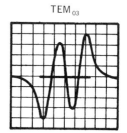

TEM$_{04}$

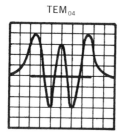

TEM$_{05}$

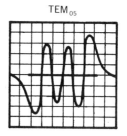

FIG. 4-9. Amplitude distributions in some low-order modes of a confocal cavity.

where $H_m(x)$ and $H_n(y)$ are Hermite polynomials, and

$$w_s = \sqrt{\frac{b\lambda}{\pi}}$$

(4-20)

is called the "spot size" of the mode. The Hermite polynomials are given by

$$H_0(\xi) = 1$$

$$H_1(\xi) = 2\xi \qquad\qquad (4\text{-}21)$$

$$H_n(\xi) = (-1)^n e^{\xi^2} \frac{d^n}{d\xi^n} e^{-\xi^2}$$

Some field distributions in low-order modes are shown in Figure 4-9, and some experimentally observed mode patterns from a gas laser are shown in Figure 4-10.

Note that the field distributions given by Eqs. (4-18) and (4-19) are independent of the size of the mirrors. This is a basic property of the modes of a confocal cavity.

Using Eq. (4-21), we find that the TEM_{00} mode of a confocal cavity has a field distribution on the mirrors of

$$u_0(x)v_0(y) = e^{-(x^2 + y^2)/w_s^2} \qquad\qquad (4\text{-}22)$$

The lowest-order mode of a confocal cavity is thus a gaussian. We see that the spot size determines the distance from the axis at which the amplitude in the TEM_{00} mode falls to $1/e$ of its axial value.

An important consequence of the Hermite-gaussian approximation for the transverse modes of a confocal cavity is that it enables one to determine the field distribution in any plane intersecting the axis of the cavity. In order to find the field distribution on a plane intersecting the axis at a distance z from the center of the cavity, one must evaluate a Fresnel integral of the general type given in Eq. (4-7). In the approximation that the modes are given by Hermite-gaussian functions, the Fresnel integral can be evaluated in closed form. Boyd and Gordon have shown that the field distribution in the TEM_{mn} mode in a plane intersecting the axis of the cavity at a distance z from its center is given by

$$u_m(x,z)v_n(y,z) = \frac{b\lambda}{\pi w_s^2} H_m\left(\frac{\sqrt{2}}{w_s}x\right) H_n\left(\frac{\sqrt{2}}{w_s}y\right) e^{-\rho^2/w_s^2} e^{-i[k(z + \rho^2/2R) + \Phi]} \qquad (4\text{-}23)$$

where

$$\rho^2 = x^2 + y^2 \qquad\qquad (4\text{-}24)$$

$$w_s = \sqrt{\frac{\lambda}{2\pi} \frac{b^2 + 4z^2}{b}} \qquad\qquad (4\text{-}25)$$

$$R = \frac{b^2 + 4z^2}{4z} \qquad\qquad (4\text{-}26)$$

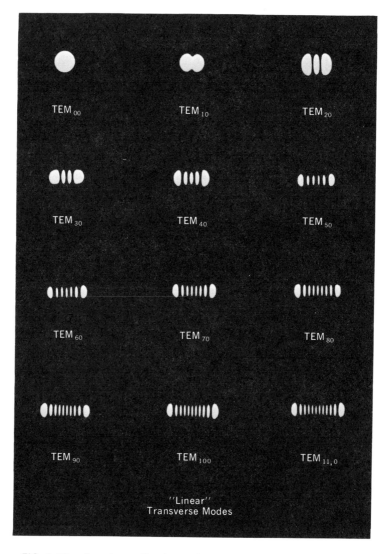

TEM$_{00}$ TEM$_{10}$ TEM$_{20}$

TEM$_{30}$ TEM$_{40}$ TEM$_{50}$

TEM$_{60}$ TEM$_{70}$ TEM$_{80}$

TEM$_{90}$ TEM$_{100}$ TEM$_{11,0}$

"Linear"
Transverse Modes

FIG. 4-10.   Experimentally observed mode patterns in some low-order modes of a confocal cavity.

and

$$\Phi = \frac{kb}{2} + (1 + m + n)\tan^{-1}\frac{b + 2z}{b - 2z} \qquad (4\text{-}27)$$

Equation (4-23) is the basic result of the Boyd and Gordon theory. It is valid at all distances z from the center of the cavity; that is, it can be used to find the field outside as well as inside the cavity.

We see from Eq. (4-25) that the quantity w_s gives the spot size at a distance z from the center of the cavity. For $z = b/2$ it reduces to its previous definition (4-20). An examination of the phase factor shows that the wavefronts are spherical near the axis and that R is equal to the radius of curvature of the wavefront at a distance z from the center of the cavity. Note that for $z = b/2$ the radius of curvature of the wavefront is b, as expected. The quantity Φ represents a phase shift which is constant across a wavefront; it amounts to a correction of the phase velocity of propagation of a mode.

The transverse modes of a confocal cavity display several interesting properties; the most important is that the "functional form" of a confocal mode is the same in *any* plane intersecting the optical axis. The spot size w_s and radius of curvature R depend, of course, on the distance z, as they must because of diffraction. However, the functional form of the field distribution is the same in any plane.

The above considerations indicate that the spot size and radius of curvature completely determine the characteristics of the modes of a confocal cavity.[3] Moreover, an examination of Eqs. (4-25) and (4-26) shows that for a given wavelength the spot size and radius of curvature at a distance z are both determined by the single parameter b. It thus follows that a knowledge of the confocal radius (and the origin $z=0$) enables one to completely determine all the transverse modes in any plane intersecting the optical axis.

It is clear that any parameter which is related to b (for example, the spot size at $z = 0$) can be used to characterize the modes of a confocal cavity. A number of different parameters have been suggested; in this book we use the confocal radius directly. Thus the spot size and radius of curvature of the transverse modes are given by Eqs. (4-25) and (4-26).

The principal advantage of using the confocal radius as the parameter characterizing the modes is that it enables one to determine the spot size and radius of curvature at any point by using simple geometrical constructions. A method for doing this, which we call the "propagation-circle method," was introduced by Deschamps and Mast, and later developed by Laures. The propagation-circle method has the disadvantage that it does not determine the spot size directly, but it has the more-than-compensating advantage that it gives a very simple visualization of the propagation of laser beams.

The quantities determined in the propagation-circle method are the radius of curvature of the wavefront, and a "beam parameter" b', which is related

---

[3] Except for the phase velocity.

to the spot size by

$$b' = \frac{\pi w_s^2}{\lambda} \qquad (4\text{-}28)$$

Introducing this into Eq. (4-25), we find an equation for the beam parameter:

$$b' = \frac{(b/2)^2 + z^2}{b/2} \qquad (4\text{-}29)$$

We may rewrite Eq. (4-26) as

$$R = \frac{(b/2)^2 + z^2}{z} \qquad (4\text{-}30)$$

These last two equations form the basis for the propagation-circle method.
Consider a confocal cavity of length b, as shown in Figure 4-11. Construct a circle σ_b centered on the point $z = 0$ having a *diameter* equal to the *radius*

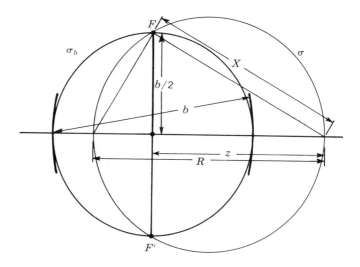

FIG. 4-11.   Construction of σ circles.

of curvature of the mirrors as shown. Construct a vertical line through the point $z = 0$, and denote the intersections of the line with the circle σ_b by F and F'. These points are called the "lateral focal points" of the confocal cavity. The distance FF' is clearly equal to the confocal radius b.

Construct a circle σ passing through the lateral focal points. The radius of curvature of a transverse mode at the point where the circle σ intersects the axis is equal to the *diameter* of the circle σ. To see this, note that

$$X^2 = \left(\frac{b}{2}\right)^2 + z^2 \tag{4-31}$$

and

$$\frac{R}{X} = \frac{X}{z} \tag{4-32}$$

Therefore,

$$R = \frac{(b/2)^2 + z^2}{z} \tag{4-33}$$

which is simply Eq. (4-30) again.

It thus follows that at any point z on the axis of a confocal cavity one can construct a circle, which we shall call a "σ circle," whose diameter is equal to the radius of curvature of the wavefront of a transverse mode of the cavity at the point z. The σ circle is defined by the requirement that it pass through the point z and the lateral focal points F and F'. Figure 4-12 shows a graphical determination of the wavefronts of the modes of a confocal cavity using σ circles.

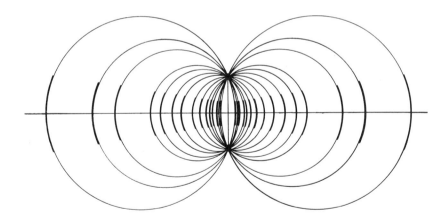

FIG. 4-12.   Wavefronts in a confocal cavity.

The beam parameter as a function of distance from the center of a confocal cavity can be determined from a different geometrical construction. Construct the circles σ_b and σ as before, and determine the lateral focal points, as shown in Figure 4-13. Now construct a circle π which passes through the lateral focal point F and is tangent to the optical axis at the point z. The

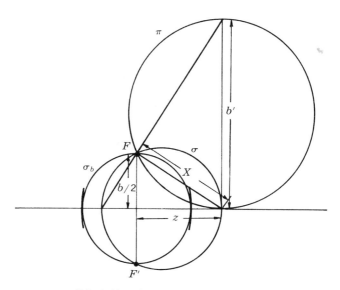

FIG. 4-13.   Construction of π circles.

diameter of the circle π is equal to the beam parameter b'. To see this, note that

$$X^2 = \left(\frac{b}{2}\right)^2 + z^2 \tag{4-34}$$

and

$$\frac{b/2}{X} = \frac{X}{b'} \tag{4-35}$$

thus

$$b' = \frac{(b/2)^2 + z^2}{b/2} \tag{4-36}$$

which is simply a restatement of Eq. (4-29).

It thus follows that at any point z on the axis of a confocal cavity one can construct a circle which we shall call a "π circle," whose diameter is equal to the beam parameter b' of a transverse mode of the cavity at the point z. The π circle is defined by the requirements that it pass through the lateral focal point F of the cavity and that it be tangent to the optical axis at the point z. The spot size w_s of the transverse mode at the distance z is determined from the beam parameter b' by the relation

$$w_s = \sqrt{\frac{b'\lambda}{\pi}} \tag{4-37}$$

The propagation-circle method forms a very simple tool for determining the propagation of Hermite-gaussian beams. Its use is not restricted to the modes of a confocal cavity, but as we shall see in the next section, it can be used to describe the modes of any curved-mirror cavity.

4-3 GENERAL CURVED-MIRROR CAVITIES

The transverse modes of a confocal cavity have wavefronts which are spherical near the optical axis of the cavity. Consider the wavefronts shown in Figure 4-12. If *any* two of the wavefronts are replaced by mirrors having the same radius of curvature as the wavefronts that they are replacing, a new cavity will be formed in the region between the two mirrors, which has the same transverse modes as those of the original confocal cavity. It thus follows that there are an infinite number of nonconfocal cavities which have the same transverse modes as those of a confocal cavity.

With any mirror of radius of curvature R, we can associate a σ circle whose *diameter* is equal to R. Consider the situation shown in Figure 4-14a, where

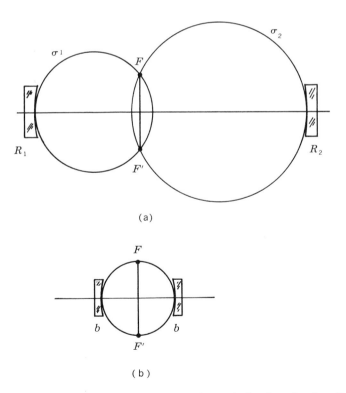

(a)

(b)

FIG. 4-14. (a) Curved-mirror cavity; (b) "equivalent" confocal cavity.

two mirrors of radius of curvature R_1 and R_2 form a nonconfocal cavity. The points F and F', where the σ circles σ_1 and σ_2 intersect, define an "equivalent" confocal cavity which will have the same transverse modes as the nonconfocal cavity. The equivalent confocal cavity corresponding to the cavity shown in Figure 4-14a is shown in Figure 4-14b.

The above considerations lead to the so-called "stability criterion" for a curved-mirror cavity: *for a curved-mirror cavity to be stable, the σ circles of the two mirrors must intersect.* If two mirrors are positioned so that their σ circles do *not* intersect, then clearly there is no equivalent confocal cavity having the same modes as the given cavity. It can be shown that in this case all the modes of the cavity have high diffraction loss. Figure 4-15 shows some examples of stable and unstable cavities.

We see from Figure 4-15a that the confocal cavity is a rather special case of a general curved-mirror cavity: it is a cavity for which the σ circles of the mirrors completely overlap. The intersection points of the σ circles are then not uniquely defined, and we could equally well take any set of points on the σ circles, such as F_1 and F_1', to define an "equivalent confocal cavity." Such a choice would give rise to transverse modes which are asymmetric in the z direction. In practice, the particular equivalent confocal cavity which has the least diffraction loss can be defined by suitably positioning an aperture stop in the cavity.

Note that the confocal cavity is unique in another respect: it is only stable if the radii of curvature of the mirrors are the same, as shown in Figure 4-15h.

One of the attractive features of the propagation-circle method for determining the stability of a general curved-mirror cavity is that not only does it indicate whether the cavity is stable but also it determines where and how big the equivalent confocal cavity is. The equivalent confocal radius can also be determined algebraically. Given a curved-mirror cavity with mirrors of radius of curvature R_1 and R_2, spaced by a distance L, we obtain for the equivalent confocal radius:

$$b = \sqrt{4d(R_1 - d)} \qquad (4\text{-}38)$$

where

$$d = \frac{L(R_2 - L)}{R_1 + R_2 - 2L} \qquad (4\text{-}39)$$

is the distance from mirror 1 to the center of the equivalent confocal cavity.

It is interesting to compare the propagation of laser modes to the propagation of light according to conventional geometrical optics. The characteristics

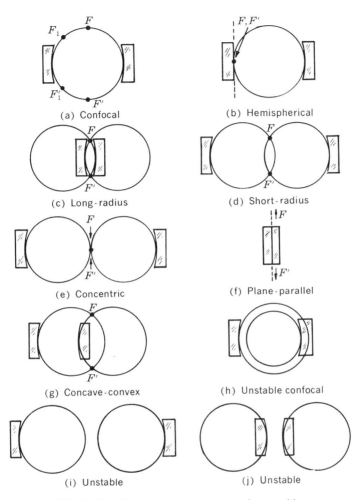

FIG. 4-15. Various types of curved-mirror cavities.

of the transverse modes of a laser are determined entirely by diffraction, so it might be thought that a laser mode would behave as though it came from a point source. An examination of Eq. (4-30) shows that such is not generally the case. Although the wavefront of a transverse mode of a curved-mirror cavity is always spherical, the apparent center of curvature depends on the distance z from the center of the equivalent confocal cavity. In the limit where the equivalent confocal radius goes to zero, however, we see from Eq. (4-30) that the radius of curvature at a point z becomes

$$R = z \qquad (4\text{-}40)$$

Hence we may conclude that the propagation of transverse modes obeys the laws of geometrical optics in the limit where the finite size of the equivalent confocal cavity can be neglected. However, note, that, according to Eq. (4-25), in this same limit the spot size goes to infinity. The Hermite-gaussian approximation then is not valid, so that the above arguments can only be taken as qualitative.

The angular divergence of a transverse mode is measured by the "far-field diffraction angle," which is defined to be the ratio of the spot size at a point z to the distance z, in the limit $z \to \infty$. From Eq. (4-25) we see that this is given by

$$\vartheta = \sqrt{\frac{2\lambda}{\pi b}} \tag{4-41}$$

It is sometimes desirable to write this last formula in terms of the spot size w_0 at the center of the equivalent confocal cavity. From Eq. (4-25), we have

$$w_0 = \sqrt{\frac{\lambda b}{2\pi}} \tag{4-42}$$

so that

$$\vartheta = \frac{\lambda}{\pi w_0} \tag{4-43}$$

Note that the field distribution of a transverse mode is most tightly concentrated at the center of the equivalent confocal cavity. The center of the equivalent confocal cavity is sometimes called the "beam waist." Note also that the angular divergence of a transverse mode is inversely proportional to the minimum spot size. The geometrical-optics approximation to laser mode propagation is thus valid when the angular divergence of the beam is large or, equivalently, when the minimum spot size is small.

4–4 CHOICE OF MIRROR CURVATURES FOR GAS-LASER CAVITIES

We have seen in the preceding section that there are a wide variety of curved-mirror cavities which have the same transverse modes as those of an equivalent confocal cavity. The choice of an optimum cavity for a particular laser depends on several factors. In this section, we shall consider some of these factors and see how they affect the choice of a cavity.

If the detailed characteristics of the output beam from a laser are of no interest (as is the case, for example, when one is looking for new laser transitions), the choice of a particular cavity is inconsequential. Any cavity which is well inside the stable region is usually satisfactory. On the other hand, if the output beam from the laser is to be used for some specific purpose, then it is usually desirable to operate the laser in the TEM_{00} transverse mode, and the optimum choice of a cavity is the cavity that maximizes the output power in the TEM_{00} mode.

The reason why it is desirable to operate lasers in the TEM_{00} mode comes from basic considerations regarding the propagation of Hermite-gaussian beams. We make the assumption that, in most applications of gas lasers, the basic objective is to obtain the maximum amount of (monochromatic) power per unit area on a surface located at a great distance from the laser.[4] If this is true, then the utility of the laser will be determined by the far-field diffraction angle of the emergent beam.

The angular divergence of the beam can be reduced to any desired value (at least in principle) by passing it through a suitable optical system. The critical quantity is the amount of power in the TEM_{00} mode. Consider any given laser cavity combined with any given optical system; the spot size of the beam at any distance from the laser is then completely determined. Since the functional form of all the transverse modes is the same in any plane intersecting the axis, the high-order transverse modes will have a greater spatial extent than the TEM_{00} mode. It follows that the amount of power per unit area will be determined by the amount of power in the TEM_{00} mode, even though the *total* output power of the laser may be greater if the laser is operated in a high-order mode.

Given a laser with a plasma tube of a certain diameter, the optimum cavity is the one having a spot size that "fills" the plasma tube. The only transverse mode having low enough loss to oscillate will then be the TEM_{00} mode, and all the output power from the laser will thus be in this mode. In practice, such a situation is obtained when the spot size is approximately one-third the diameter of the plasma tube.

The diameter of the plasma tube for a given laser is often determined by spectroscopic considerations. For example, in a neutral-spectrum gas laser, the gain coefficient is observed to vary inversely with the plasma-tube diameter. Thus, as will be shown in Chapter 6, the output *intensity* of a neutral-spectrum laser increases as the plasma-tube diameter is reduced. On the other hand, the output *power* of a laser increases as the square of the plasma-tube diameter, if the gain coefficient remains constant. There is thus an optimum diameter

---

[4] This is equivalent to obtaining the maximum amount of power in the focus of a lens.

for the plasma tube at which the increase in output power due to the area factor balances the decrease in output power due to the reduction in the gain coefficient. Once this diameter is found, the optimum cavity is determined to be the one having a spot size approximately equal to one-third of this diameter. In a typical gas laser, the usual problem is to find a cavity having a spot size sufficiently large to fill the plasma-tube diameter.

Figure 4-16 shows a plot of the spot sizes in a cavity comprising one plane mirror and one curved mirror, as a function of the radius of curvature of the

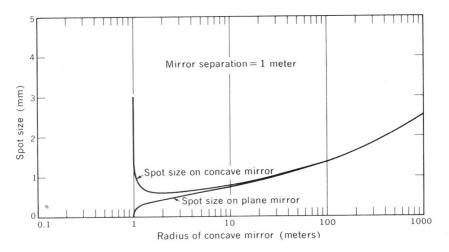

FIG. 4-16. Spot sizes versus radius of concave mirror in a plano-concave cavity.

curved mirror. The spot size on the curved mirror is seen to increase as the cavity approaches either a hemispherical or plane-parallel (long-radius) configuration. It is usually desirable to use one or the other of these configurations.

The choice between a hemispherical and a long-radius cavity depends on the diameter of the plasma tube. For large-diameter plasma tubes, the long-radius cavity becomes very difficult to align, and the hemispherical cavity is the best choice, although the mode "volume" in a hemispherical cavity has a maximum fractional value of only one-third, since the spot size on the plane mirror approaches zero in the hemispherical limit. For small-diameter plasma tubes, the larger mode volume of the long-radius cavity makes it the optimum choice. The crossover point in practical lasers seems to be when the Fresnel number of the cavity is in the range from 5 to 10.

4–5   RESONANCE CONDITIONS IN GENERAL CURVED-MIRROR CAVITIES

We have seen in Section 4–3 that for any stable curved-mirror cavity there is an equivalent confocal cavity which has the same transverse modes as does the general cavity. The equivalence of the two cavities only pertains to the spot sizes and radii of curvature of the transverse modes. Since the two cavities are of different lengths, the resonant frequencies of the longitudinal modes will be different. Moreover, because of the presence of the phase factor Φ in Eq. (4-23), the transverse modes of a general curved-mirror cavity will not possess the high degree of degeneracy possessed by the modes of a confocal cavity. The resonance condition for a mode of a general curved-mirror cavity can be written as

$$\Omega = \frac{\pi c}{L}\left[q + \frac{1}{\pi}(1 + m + n)\cos^{-1}\sqrt{\left(1 - \frac{L}{R_1}\right)\left(1 - \frac{L}{R_2}\right)}\right] \quad (4\text{-}44)$$

where R_1 and R_2 are the radii of curvature of the mirrors, and L is their separation.

We see from Eq. (4-44) that the transverse mode resonances for a general curved-mirror cavity depend on the order numbers of the modes. Thus, for example, the TEM$_{00}$ mode will in general resonate at a different frequency than the TEM$_{20}$ mode. However, note that, if $R_1 = R_2 = L$, the resonance condition reduces to that given by Eq. (4-17) for a confocal cavity, and the TEM$_{00}$ and TEM$_{20}$ modes have the same set of resonance frequencies.

Note that if

$$\cos^{-1}\sqrt{\left(1 - \frac{L}{R_1}\right)\left(1 - \frac{L}{R_2}\right)} = \frac{\pi}{l} \quad (4\text{-}45)$$

where l is an integer, then the resonance condition (4-44) can be written as

$$\Omega = \frac{\pi c}{lL}[lq + 1 + m + n] \quad (4\text{-}46)$$

In this case, since increasing the sum $(m + n)$ by l and decreasing q by 1 leaves the resonant frequency unchanged, there will be l sets of degenerate transverse modes of the cavity. The confocal cavity is a simple example of the general degeneracy condition (4-45), corresponding to $l = 2$. Cavities which satisfy Eq. (4-45) are said to be "mode-degenerate," or "reentrant," cavities; it can be shown that a ray launched in such a cavity will retrace its path after l complete traversals.

4–6 PROPAGATION-CIRCLE METHODS FOR GAUSSIAN BEAMS

Practically all applications of gas lasers involve sending the beam through some sort of optical system. In this section, we shall consider the general way in which laser beams behave when they are transmitted through such optical systems. We shall assume that we are dealing with a laser beam emitted from a curved-mirror cavity in the TEM_{00} transverse mode.

For the most part, we shall assume that all the optical elements in optical systems have diameters which are larger than the laser beam diameter, so that we need not consider the diffraction effects caused by "truncating" the gaussian amplitude distribution. Under this assumption the field distribution in any plane perpendicular to the axis of propagation is gaussian.

It is perhaps appropriate to note at this point that the propagation of gaussian beams through *weak* focusing systems is slightly different from what one might expect on the basis of purely geometrical considerations. If the focusing system is strong, so that the angles of convergence and divergence of the beam are large, then ordinary geometrical optics is adequate to treat the problem. We shall consider first the exact propagation laws for a gaussian beam, and then show how geometrical optics appears as a limiting case for beams having larger convergence or divergence angles.

We shall neglect any consideration of the aberrations of optical systems.

The most common parameters used to characterize a gaussian beam are its spot size and radius of curvature. As described in Section 4-2, it is expedient not to use the spot size of the beam in direct calculations, but rather the beam parameter, which is related to the spot size as follows:

$$b' = \frac{\pi w_s^2}{\lambda} \tag{4-47}$$

If we know the beam parameter and radius of curvature of a gaussian beam at one point, we can find the beam parameter and radius of curvature at any other point by using the propagation-circle method described in Section 4-2.

Suppose the beam parameter and radius of curvature have values b_0' and R_0 at some point z_0. We associate with the beam parameter a π circle π_0 whose diameter is equal to b_0', and we associate with the radius of curvature a σ circle σ_0 whose diameter is equal to R_0, as shown in Figure 4-17. According to the analysis of Section 4-2, the circle σ_0 and the circle π_0 must intersect at the lateral focal point F. Since the propagation of a gaussian beam is completely determined by the location of its lateral focal points, we can find the beam parameter and radius of curvature at any other point z_1 by constructing new σ and π circles which pass through F and z_1.

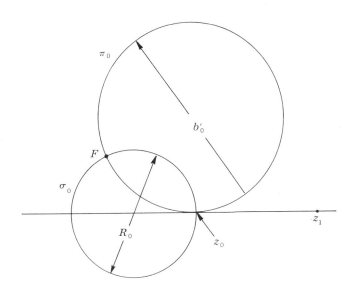

FIG. 4-17.   Determination of the lateral focal points of a gaussian beam.

Up to this point in the discussion we have used the concept of propagation circles to describe the propagation of a gaussian beam in free space. It is easy to extend the concept to describe the propagation of a gaussian beam through an optical system. We may begin by considering propagation through a thin lens.

A beam of radius of curvature R_1 entering a thin lens of focal length f is transformed into a beam of radius of curvature R_2 leaving the thin lens, where R_1 and R_2 are related by the thin-lens equation,

$$\frac{1}{R_2} - \frac{1}{R_1} = \frac{1}{f} \tag{4-48}$$

If the lens is thin, the diameter of the beam is not changed in passing through it.

Consider a gaussian beam incident on a thin lens L having a focal length f, as shown in Figure 4-18. Let the incident beam be characterized by lateral focal points F_0 and F_0' as shown. The beam parameter and radius of curvature of the beam incident on the lens can then be characterized by the propagation circles σ_0 and π_0 as shown.

Since the lens will alter the radius of curvature of the beam according to Eq. (4-48), the beam emerging from the lens will be characterized by a new σ circle, σ_1. The σ circle σ_1 is defined by the requirement that it intersect the axis at the vertex of the lens and at the point A_1 shown in Figure 4-18. The point A_1 is the geometrical image of the point A_0 formed by the lens. Since a thin lens does not alter the beam parameter, the emergent beam will be characterized by the same π circle π_0 as the incident beam.

The beam emerging from the thin lens L is thus characterized by the propagation circles σ_1 and π_0. The point where these circles intersect determines the lateral focal point F_1 of the emergent beam. Once the new lateral focal point is found, the propagation of the beam after it passes through the lens is completely determined.

We see from Figure 4-18 that the minimum spot size of the emergent beam, or the "beam waist," is always closer to the lens than the geometrical focus. That is, the minimum spot size occurs at the point B_1, where the line $F_1 F_1'$ intersects the optical axis; whereas the geometrical focus is at the point A_1.

The minimum spot size of the emergent beam is

$$w_0 = \sqrt{\frac{b_1' \lambda}{2\pi}} \tag{4-49}$$

where b_1' is the length of the line $F_1 F_1'$ (that is, b_1' is the new "equivalent confocal radius" of the beam).

Figure 4-18 indicates when the geometrical-optics approximation is valid: the geometrical-optics approximation is valid when the two lateral focal

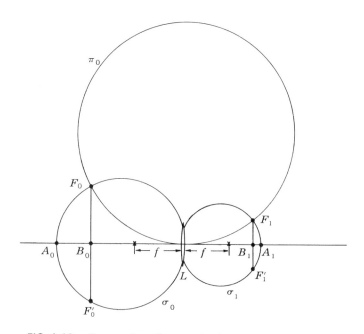

FIG. 4-18.   Propagation of a gaussian beam through a thin lens.

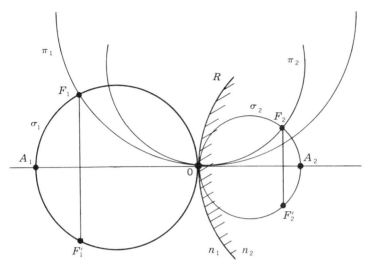

FIG. 4-19. Propagation of a gaussian beam through a spherical interface.

points F_1 and F_1' merge at the point A_1. This will occur when the propagation circle π_0 is large: that is, when the spot size of the beam on the lens is large.

The propagation-circle method described above can also be used to determine the propagation of gaussian beams through an interface between materials having different refractive indices. Consider the situation shown in Figure 4-19. We have a surface of radius of curvature R which separates media of refractive index n_1 and n_2. Suppose that in medium 1 we have a gaussian beam characterized by a lateral focal point F_1. At the refracting interface the beam can thus be characterized by propagation circles σ_1 and π_1 as shown. The refracting interface alters the radius of curvature of the wavefront according to the standard formula:

$$\frac{n_2}{R_2} + \frac{n_1}{R_1} = \frac{n_2 - n_1}{R} \tag{4-50}$$

where R_1 and R_2 are the radii of curvature in media 1 and 2. It thus follows that the propagation circle σ_2 is defined by the requirement that it pass through the points 0 and A_2, where A_2 is the geometrical image of A_1 determined by Eq. (4-50).

In order to determine the propagation circle π_2, we must generalize the discussion given for the case of a thin lens. In particular, we have in general that the *optical* length of the beam parameter remains constant as the beam traverses the interface between two refracting media. It thus follows that the beam parameter b_2' at the interface is related to the beam parameter b_1' at the interface as follows:

$$b_2' = \frac{n_1}{n_2} b_1' \qquad (4\text{-}51)$$

The propagation circle π_2 thus has a diameter which is n_1/n_2 times the diameter of π_1.

The lateral focal point F_2 is determined by the intersection of the propagation circles σ_2 and π_2; once F_2 is found, the propagation of the beam in medium 2 is completely determined.

A common problem in gas-laser technology involves "matching" the transverse modes from one cavity into another. This problem can be conveniently solved by using propagation circles. Suppose that we have two cavities as shown in Figure 4-20. The lateral focus of one cavity is F_1, and the

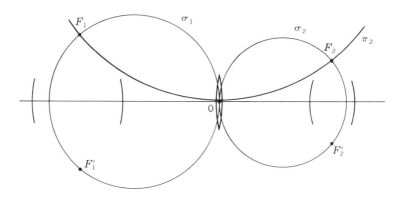

FIG. 4-20.   "Mode matching" two cavities.

lateral focus of the other cavity is F_2. The modes of the two cavities can be matched by putting a thin lens at position 0 as shown. The position 0 is determined by constructing the π circle which is tangent to the axis and passes through F_1 and F_2. The point where the π circle touches the axis is the proper location for the lens. The required focal length of the lens can be determined by constructing the σ circles σ_1 and σ_2 to determine the radii of curvature of the wavefronts from the two cavities at the point 0. These radii of curvature can then be inserted in the thin-lens equation (4-48) to determine the required focal length.

It should be mentioned that, if the cavity mirrors have plane back surfaces and curved reflecting surfaces, then the mirrors will act as negative lenses. If accurate mode matching is necessary, this fact should be taken into account.

4–7 ALGEBRAIC METHODS FOR GAUSSIAN BEAMS

Although the propagation-circle method described in the preceding section is useful for visualizing the propagation of gaussian beams through optical systems, often it is either insufficiently accurate or too cumbersome to use for calculations. In such cases, it is desirable to work directly with the algebraic expressions for the spot size and radius of curvature:

$$w_s{}^2 = \frac{\lambda}{\pi} \left[\frac{(b/2)^2 + z^2}{b/2} \right] \qquad (4\text{-}52)$$

and

$$R = \frac{(b/2)^2 + z^2}{z} \qquad (4\text{-}53)$$

As noted before, these equations give a complete description of the propagation of gaussian beams. In many practical situations, however, it is not convenient to work with the equivalent confocal radius; a more useful parameter is the spot size at the beam waist, w_0, which is related to b by

$$w_0 = \sqrt{\frac{b\lambda}{2\pi}} \qquad (4\text{-}54)$$

Using this equation in (4-52) and (4-53), we find that

$$w_s{}^2 = w_0{}^2 \left[1 + \left(\frac{\lambda z}{\pi w_0{}^2} \right)^2 \right] \qquad (4\text{-}55)$$

and

$$R = z \left[1 + \left(\frac{\pi w_0{}^2}{\lambda z} \right)^2 \right] \qquad (4\text{-}56)$$

These last equations are particularly useful for finding the spot size and radius of curvature at a distance z from a collimator. A beam leaving a collimator has a plane wavefront as it leaves the collimator, so that the lateral focal points of the beam are located in the plane of the collimator objective. The waist of the emergent beam is consequently located in this plane, and the spot size of the emergent beam corresponds to w_0. Equations (4-55) and (4-56) thus enable one to compute the spot size and radius of curvature at any distance z measured from the plane of the collimator objective.

It is often desirable to invert Eqs. (4-55) and (4-56) to find the minimum spot size and the location of the beam waist in terms of w_s and R. We have

$$w_0{}^2 = \frac{w_s{}^2}{1 + (\pi w_s{}^2/\lambda R)^2} \tag{4-57}$$

and

$$z = \frac{R}{1 + (\lambda R/\pi w_s{}^2)^2} \tag{4-58}$$

These last formulas are useful for determining the characteristics of a gaussian beam which has been focused by a lens. Thus if we know the spot size and the radius of curvature of a beam as it leaves a lens, we can find the position of the focus and the spot size at the focus by using Eqs. (4-57) and (4-58).

The above formulas can be simplified if the angle of convergence or divergence of the beam is large. The far-field diffraction angle of the beam is

$$\vartheta = \frac{\lambda}{\pi w_0} \tag{4-59}$$

which can be written with the aid of Eq. (4-57) as

$$\vartheta = \frac{w_0}{z} \frac{\pi w_s{}^2}{\lambda R} \tag{4-60}$$

Assuming that $\vartheta \gg w_0/z$, we can thus write Eqs. (4-57) and (4-58) as

$$w_s = \vartheta z \tag{4-61}$$

and

$$R = z \tag{4-62}$$

These last expressions correspond to the geometrical-optics approximation.

In the geometrical-optics approximation it is often convenient to characterize a beam by its f number, which is defined by

$$f^{\#} \equiv \frac{1}{2\vartheta} = \frac{\pi w_0}{2\lambda} \tag{4-63}$$

This last equation gives a very convenient expression for the minimum spot size in the focus of a lens. We have

$$w_0 = \frac{2}{\pi} \lambda f^{\#} \tag{4-64}$$

The formulas given above provide a useful method for calculating the propagation of gaussian beams through optical systems. Several alternate methods, which we shall not consider, have been developed: Kogelnik, for example, has developed a matrix method for determining the propagation of gaussian beams through optical systems, and Collins has developed a method using "circle diagrams" which is somewhat analogous to the propagation-circle method described in Section 4-2.

4–8 SPECIAL TOPICS CONCERNING TRANSVERSE MODES

There are a number of topics relating to transverse mode structure in optical cavities which should be mentioned but which cannot be discussed in detail, either because of space limitations or because they have not yet been fully investigated. In this section we shall consider some of these topics.

Most gas lasers employ curved-mirror cavities of the type described in Section 4–3. There are, however, several other types of cavities which are occasionally used and thereby warrant mention.

There are several different types of laser cavities which use more than two mirrors for longitudinal mode selection; these cavities will be described in detail in the next chapter. Multiple-mirror cavities are also used in "ring" lasers. A typical ring-laser cavity is shown in Figure 4-21a. Such a cavity has properties similar to those of an ordinary curved-mirror cavity, except that the curved mirror will display astigmatism, since it is used off-axis. The stability criterion for a cavity such as that shown in Figure 4-21a is that the radius of curvature of the curved mirror be greater than one-half the perimeter of the resonator.

In infrared gas lasers, particularly the CO_2 laser, it is common practice to use a "hole-coupled" cavity such as that shown in Figure 4-21b. The purpose of the hole is, of course, to enable light to pass through an otherwise opaque mirror. The hole-coupled cavity is thus useful for those parts of the spectrum where partially transmitting mirrors are not available.

A cavity somewhat related to the hole-coupled cavity is the unstable cavity shown in Figure 4-21c. In an unstable cavity, use is made of the large diffraction loss to provide output coupling for the beam. The unstable cavity should have good mode discrimination, but it has not yet been investigated in detail.

In Section 4–2 it was shown that the modes of a confocal cavity could be approximated by Hermite-gaussian functions. The Hermite-gaussian functions are applicable to a cavity having rectangular symmetry. For a system

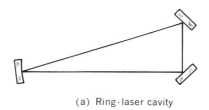

(a) Ring-laser cavity

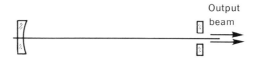

(b) Hole-coupled cavity

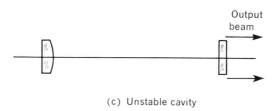

(c) Unstable cavity

FIG. 4-21.   Special laser cavities: (a) ring-laser cavity; (b) hole-coupled cavity; (c) unstable cavity.

having cylindrical symmetry, the transverse modes are given by

$$u_l(\rho,\varphi) = \left(\sqrt{2}\,\frac{\rho}{w_s}\right)^l L_p^l\left(2\,\frac{\rho^2}{w_s^2}\right)e^{-\rho^2/w_s^2}e^{-i\{k[z+(\rho^2/2R)]+l\varphi+\Phi\}} \qquad (4\text{-}65)$$

where

$$\rho^2 = x^2 + y^2 \qquad (4\text{-}66)$$

$$w_s = \sqrt{\frac{\lambda}{2\pi}\,\frac{b^2+4z^2}{b}} \qquad (4\text{-}67)$$

$$R = \frac{b^2+4z^2}{4z} \qquad (4\text{-}68)$$

$$\Phi = \frac{kb}{2} + (1+2p+l)\tan^{-1}\frac{b+2z}{b-2z} \qquad (4\text{-}69)$$

and L_p^l is an associated Laguerre polynomial; p and l are the radial and angular mode numbers. The first two associated Laguerre polynomials are

$$L_0{}^l\left(2\,\frac{\rho^2}{w_s{}^2}\right) = 1 \tag{4-70}$$

$$L_1{}^l\left(2\,\frac{\rho^2}{w_s{}^2}\right) = l + 1 - 2\,\frac{\rho^2}{w_s{}^2} \tag{4-71}$$

We see from Eqs. (4-65) and (4-70) that the TEM_{00} mode in cylindrical coordinates is a gaussian, as it is in cartesian coordinates.

So far, in the discussion of this chapter, we have considered the transverse mode structure of *passive* cavities. The transverse mode structure of *active* cavities has been studied by Fox and Li. Their analysis shows that the transverse modes of an active cavity are very nearly the same as those of a passive cavity. One of the interesting results of the Fox and Li study is that the modes of a plane-parallel cavity behave in a somewhat different manner from those of a confocal cavity: In a plane-parallel cavity, the TEM_{00} mode is always the favored mode, but in a confocal cavity the mode having the highest loss not exceeding the gain is the favored mode.

The Fox and Li analysis of the transverse modes of an active cavity assumes that the modes are tuned to the center of the atomic transition, so that there can be no radial variation of the refractive index of the gas. If the modes are not tuned to the center of the atomic transition, there will be saturation effects in the refractive index which will tend to focus modes oscillating on the low-frequency side of line center and defocus modes oscillating on the high-frequency side of line center. Thus gas lasers should show some tendency to oscillate on the low-frequency side of the atomic transition, because of reduced diffraction losses. This effect has not yet been investigated in detail. It is apparently a small effect in a normal gas laser, and the Fox and Li study seems adequate to explain existing experimental data.

The output beam from many gas lasers, particularly ones using long-radius-mirror cavities, does not have a gaussian amplitude distribution, even when the laser is operated in the TEM_{00} transverse mode. The reason for this is that the walls of the plasma tube normally constitute the aperture stop of the cavity. Light diffracted out of the mode reflects off the walls of the plasma tube, and if the angle of incidence is sufficiently close to grazing, this light may appear in the output beam of the laser.

The extraneous light in the beam can be eliminated by passing the beam through a device called a "spatial filter." The spatial filter consists of two lenses having a common focus and a pinhole placed at the focus, as shown in

Figure 4-22. The diameter of the pinhole is on the order of four times the spot size at the focus of the lens. Light coming from the laser in the TEM_{00} mode thus passes through the pinhole with negligible loss, but extraneous light reflected off the walls of the plasma tube is not focused on the pinhole and is consequently eliminated from the beam.

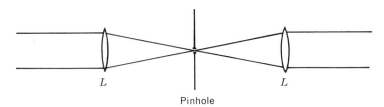

Pinhole

FIG. 4-22.   A "spatial filter."

REFERENCES

1. G. D. Boyd and J. P. Gordon, *Bell Syst. Tech. J.*, **40**: 489 (1961); G. D. Boyd and H. Kogelnik, *Bell Syst. Tech. J.*, **41**: 1347 (1962).

These two papers, along with the 1961 Fox and Li paper cited below, are the standard papers on laser mode structure. The above two papers describe the analytic solution for the modes of curved-mirror cavities.

2. A. G. Fox and T. Li, *Bell Syst. Tech. J.*, **40**: 453 (1961); A. G. Fox and T. Li, *Proc. IEEE*, **51**: 80 (1963); A. G. Fox and T. Li, *IEEE J. Quantum Electronics*, **QE-2**: 774 (1966).

   The first of these papers describes the modes of both plane-parallel and confocal cavities, using a method employing Huygens' principle and numerical analysis. This approach, although it is not so elegant as the Boyd and Gordon approach, is considerably more flexible. The last two papers extend the work to include cavities with alignment errors and cavities containing amplifying materials.

3. G. A. Deschamps and P. E. Mast, in "Proceedings of the Symposium on Quasi-Optics," p. 379, Polytechnic Press, New York, 1964; P. Laures, *Appl. Optics*, **6**: 747 (1967).

These papers describe the "propagation-circle method" for gaussian-beam analysis.

4. H. Kogelnik and T. Li, *Appl. Optics*, **5**: 1550 (1966).

This is a good review paper on laser mode structure.

5. R. L. Fork, D. R. Herriott, and H. Kogelnik, *Appl. Optics*, **3**: 1471 (1964).

Although this paper is primarily devoted to a discussion of spherical-mirror interferometers, it also contains a good discussion of transverse mode structure, particularly of those aspects which relate to mode matching.

5 LONGITUDINAL-MODE STRUCTURE

The output beam from an "ideal" laser would consist of a single transverse mode and a single longitudinal mode. Such a beam would be, for all practical purposes, completely coherent.

It was seen in Chapter 4 that it is fairly easy to constrain a laser to operate in a single transverse mode: by judiciously choosing the laser cavity, the diffraction losses for the various transverse modes can be raised to the point where only the lowest-order mode can oscillate.

It is also fairly easy to constrain a laser to operate in a single longitudinal mode. By making the laser sufficiently short, the cavity resonance frequencies can be spaced far enough apart so that there is only one cavity resonance on which amplification can occur. However, this method for obtaining single-frequency operation of a gas laser is not entirely satisfactory: the required cavity length is usually so short that the output power of the laser is severely limited.

Fortunately, it is possible to construct long lasers which only oscillate in a single longitudinal mode; in fact, it is even possible to obtain single-frequency outputs from lasers which oscillate in several longitudinal modes.

In this chapter we shall describe some of the techniques which have been suggested for obtaining high-power single-frequency output beams from gas lasers. All the schemes described in this chapter have been demonstrated experimentally.

Because of the rapidity with which this aspect of gas-laser technology is advancing, we shall not attempt to describe the current state of the art in great detail but shall confine our discussion to a general consideration of the problems involved in obtaining single-frequency output beams from gas lasers.

5-1   SINGLE-LONGITUDINAL-MODE LASERS

As mentioned above, the simplest way to obtain a single-frequency output from a gas laser is to constrain the laser so that it only oscillates in a single longitudinal mode. There are several ways to do this; in this section we shall consider two.

The most common method is to make the laser sufficiently short that there is only one cavity resonance within the Doppler width of the laser transition. This method is reliable; but as mentioned above, for many laser transitions the required length of the cavity is so short that the available output power is severely limited. For the helium-neon 6328-Å transition, the maximum possible length of the cavity is 10 to 15 cm; the maximum output power

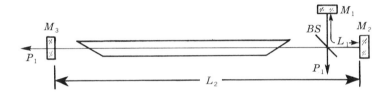

FIG. 5-1.   Fox-Smith interferometer used as a longitudinal mode selector.

of such a laser is a few milliwatts. For ion laser transitions the required lengths are considerably shorter (~ 3 cm), and the maximum output power is again a few milliwatts. In the CO_2 laser the situation is considerably improved: it is possible to use cavities having lengths on the order of 1 m, and single-frequency output powers of several watts can be obtained.

It is possible to constrain the oscillation in a long laser to a single longitudinal mode by constructing the cavity in such a manner that it only has a high quality factor for one longitudinal mode within the Doppler width of the laser transition. A common method for doing this employs a device called a "Fox-Smith interferometer."

The Fox-Smith interferometer is illustrated in Figure 5-1. It consists of two mirrors M_1 and M_2 and a beam splitter BS. The reflectance of the mirrors should be as close to unity as possible.

The reflectance versus wavelength characteristic of a Fox-Smith interferometer is identical to the transmittance versus wavelength characteristic of a Fabry-Perot interferometer. Assume, for the moment, that the mirrors M_1 and M_2 have a reflectance of unity and that losses in the beam splitter and the mirrors can be neglected. Then, if the interferometer is resonant, all the light entering the interferometer will be reflected back on itself, regardless of the reflectance of the beam splitter. The effect of changing the reflectance of the beam splitter is to change the Q of the interferometer.

The Fox-Smith interferometer can be used as one mirror of a conventional two-mirror laser cavity, as shown in Figure 5-1. To constrain the laser so that it only oscillates in a single longitudinal mode, the length L_1 should be chosen so that the interferometer has only one resonance frequency within the amplification bandwidth of the laser transition. The length L_2 of the cavity formed by the mirrors M_2 and M_3 is determined by the requirement that the long and short cavities have a common resonance frequency within this bandwidth, as illustrated in Figure 5-2.

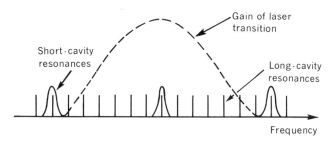

FIG. 5-2. Resonance in a single-frequency laser employing a Fox-Smith interferometer.

The principal difficulty in using a Fox-Smith interferometer as a longitudinal mode selector is that the long and short cavities must be simultaneously resonant, which means that the lengths L_1 and L_2 must be stabilized to a small fraction of a wavelength. It is possible, however, to build a servosystem which "locks" the length L_2 to the length L_1.

When the cavities L_1 and L_2 are slightly detuned, the simple reflectance argument given above is not fully adequate to explain the operation of the laser, for one must also consider the phase shift of the mode upon reflecting from the interferometer. The effect of the phase shift is that, for small detuning, the longitudinal mode defined by the cavity L_2 is "pulled" toward the longitudinal mode defined by the cavity L_1.

In a practical longitudinal mode selector using a Fox-Smith interferometer, it is not feasible to use a high-reflectance beam splitter, because scattering losses in the mirrors and beam splitter severely limit the maximum reflectance of the interferometer; beam-splitter reflectances of 30 to 60 percent are typically employed. Under these conditions, there is usually more than one longitudinal mode of the cavity L_2 which "sees" a moderately high reflectance from the interferometer. To determine the exact value of the reflectance seen by such a mode, it is necessary to take into account the frequency-pulling effects described above.

It is important that the transverse modes of the cavity L_1 be matched to the transverse modes of the cavity L_2. Such mode matching can be achieved by the proper selection of the radii of curvature of the mirrors M_1, M_2, and M_3. The transverse modes of the two cavities will be matched if the lateral focal points of the two cavities are coincident, and the matching requirements can be easily determined by using the techniques described in Chapter 4.

Two special configurations are worthy of mention. The first uses flat mirrors for both M_1 and M_2 and a long-radius mirror for M_3. Although the cavities in this case are not strictly mode-matched, the deviation from matching is essentially negligible. In the second configuration, the cavity L_2 defined by M_2 and M_3 is made confocal. The mirror M_1 is then either long-radius or flat. This configuration works by exciting an asymmetric mode of the confocal cavity L_2, as described in Chapter 4; the particular asymmetric mode which is excited depends on the radius of curvature of M_3 and the cavity length L_1. The principal advantage of this configuration is that the cavity length L_1 is not critical; the same set of mirrors can be used for a variety of interferometer lengths.

5–2 PHASE-LOCKED LASERS

In a normal multimode laser having free-running longitudinal modes, the relative phases of the various modes will be essentially random functions of time. The coherence length of the light from the laser will then be determined by the overall linewidth of the laser transition. In particular, one can show that the coherence length Δz is given by

$$\Delta z \approx \frac{2\pi c}{\Delta \omega} \qquad (5\text{-}1)$$

where c is the velocity of light, and $\Delta \omega$ is the oscillation bandwidth of the laser. The coherence length given by Eq. (5-1) is approximately the coherence length of the spontaneous emission emitted on the laser transition. A multimode laser with free-running modes thus has no advantages over an "ordinary" light source with respect to coherence length; the only advantage of the laser is that it has a higher degree of spatial coherence.

On the other hand, if the various longitudinal modes of a multimode laser are locked in phase, the coherence properties of the output beam are, in many respects, more like those of a single-frequency laser than those of an ordinary light source.

There is, in fact, a basic similarity between a multimode phase-locked laser and a single-frequency laser: A multimode phase-locked laser beam is formally equivalent to a single-frequency beam which has been pulse-modulated at the difference frequency between adjacent longitudinal modes. By using a suitable "demodulator," it is, in principle, possible to convert a phase-locked multimode beam to a single-frequency beam.

Techniques for obtaining phase-locked operation of multimode gas lasers are consequently of great interest. In this section, we shall consider some of the techniques which have been suggested and some general characteristics of phase-locked multimode oscillations.

One instance of phase locking, which we may call "self-locking," has been described in Chapter 3. If the longitudinal modes of a three-mode laser are symmetrically located with respect to the center frequency of the laser transition, then the relative phase angle [see Eq. (3-65)] will be constant in time, so that the frequency differences $\omega_2 - \omega_1$ and $\omega_3 - \omega_2$ will be exactly equal. If the phase angle φ_3 is equal to the phase angle φ_1, the oscillation in the laser is entirely equivalent to a single-frequency signal at ω_2 which is amplitude-modulated at the difference frequency $\omega_2 - \omega_1 = \omega_3 - \omega_2$. That is, in a three-mode phase-locked laser, the outer modes can be regarded as "sidebands," and the central mode can be regarded as a "carrier."

It is possible to obtain self-locking in lasers which oscillate simultaneously in more than three longitudinal modes. The effect is more difficult to obtain, however, because of the nonlinear power-independent frequency pulling described in Chapter 3. If only three modes of the laser are excited, when the modes are symmetrically located with respect to line center, the difference frequency $\omega_2 - \omega_1$ will be approximately equal to $\omega_3 - \omega_2$, even when the modes are free-running. On the other hand, if there are, for example, five modes symmetrically located with respect to line center, the difference frequencies between the "outer" adjacent modes will not coincide with the difference frequencies between "inner" adjacent modes. The combination tones which drive the modes will then be polychromatic, and a steady-state solution for the mode amplitudes and frequencies will, in general, not exist. Under certain circumstances it is possible to make one "set" of combination tones dominate and thereby to obtain self-locking of a multimode laser, but in general it is desirable to "induce" phase locking by "artificial" techniques.

The longitudinal modes of a gas laser can be locked in phase by introducing into the laser cavity a loss or phase perturbation at the difference frequency between adjacent longitudinal modes.

Suppose that a loss modulator (for example, an ultrasonic diffraction grating) is placed inside a multimode laser cavity and that it is adjusted so that it varies the cavity loss at a frequency equal to the difference frequency between adjacent longitudinal modes. The effect of the modulator on the longitudinal modes will be to produce sidebands on the modes which have frequencies corresponding to the frequencies of the adjacent longitudinal modes. The sidebands will have a definite phase relation to the carrier: it can be shown that $\varphi_{k+1} - \varphi_k = \pi$.

If the sidebands generated by the modulator are strong enough so that they constitute the main "driving" terms for the modes, the modes will phase-lock to one another.

For a short laser, the amount of sideband power required is primarily determined by the nonlinear frequency pulling in the laser, whereas for a long laser the amount of sideband power required is primarily determined by the combination tones generated within the laser. In order that the required sideband power be minimized, the laser should be short enough so that the spacing between adjacent longitudinal modes is greater than the homogeneous linewidth, but not too much shorter.

The position of the modulator in the cavity determines the amount of coupling which can be obtained between different longitudinal modes. The reason for this is apparent from the same considerations which led to the definition of "spatial Fourier components" of the inversion density in Chapter 3: namely, one must take into account the standing-wave fields of the different longitudinal modes. By using the same arguments as we used in Chapter 3, one can show that the maximum amount of coupling between adjacent longitudinal modes will occur when the modulator is located at one end of the laser cavity.

If there are several longitudinal modes excited in the laser, the output beam will take the form of a periodic pulse train. To see this, note that, if all the modes have equal amplitudes E_0, then the total field in the laser can be written as

$$E_T = E_0 \, [\cos \omega t - \cos (\omega - \Delta)t - \cos (\omega + \Delta)t$$
$$+ \cos (\omega - 2\,\Delta)t + \cos (\omega + 2\,\Delta)t - \cdots] \quad (5\text{-}2)$$

or

$$E_T = E_0 \cos \omega t \, [1 - 2 \cos \Delta t + 2 \cos 2\,\Delta t - \cdots] \quad (5\text{-}3)$$

where $\Delta \approx \pi c/L$ is the frequency difference between adjacent longitudinal modes. The series in Eq. (5-3) can be summed in closed form. If there are $(2N + 1)$ modes, we find that

$$E_T = \left[\frac{\sin (N + 1)\,\Delta t + \sin N\,\Delta t}{\sin \Delta t} \right] E_0 \cos \omega t \quad (5\text{-}4)$$

The quantity in brackets in this expression corresponds to a pulse having a "height" $= 2N + 1$, a "width" $\approx 3/N$, and a repetition frequency Δ. We thus see that an AM phase-locked oscillation can be regarded as a pulse-modulated single-frequency signal.

It is important to note that in an "ideal" situation the introduction of a loss perturbation in a laser cavity does not actually result in there being any loss for the laser oscillation. We have seen that if there are a large number of AM phase-locked modes oscillating in the cavity, the total field takes the form of a short pulse which bounces back and forth between the mirrors. It can be shown that the pulse passes through the modulator at the instant when its attenuation is zero, so that in the limit of an infinitesimally short pulse, there is no loss introduced by the modulator. It thus follows that, to a first approximation, the process of phase locking the modes of a laser by loss modulation does not change the average output power of the laser.

On the other hand, the peak output power of an AM phase-locked laser can be considerably greater than the average output power. One can easily show that the ratio of the peak output power to the average output power is approximately equal to the number of phase-locked modes and that the half-power pulse width is approximately equal to the reciprocal of the oscillation bandwidth of the laser. An AM phase-locked laser is consequently an attractive light source for applications where high peak powers are needed (for example, in systems using nonlinear effects).

As mentioned above, it is also possible to induce phase locking in a laser by introducing into the laser cavity a phase perturbation (using, for example, an electrooptic crystal) at the difference frequency between adjacent longitudinal modes. The nature of the phase-locked signal obtained by using a phase perturbation depends critically on the frequency of the perturbation.

If the perturbation frequency is exactly equal to the difference frequency between adjacent longitudinal modes, the modes will phase-lock as described above; that is, the total field will be a pulse-modulated signal. However, if the perturbation frequency is sufficiently detuned from the difference frequency between adjacent longitudinal modes (typically by about one part per thousand), the various longitudinal modes will phase-lock with Bessel-function relative amplitudes (so that the upper sidebands will be out of phase with the lower sidebands). The multimode oscillation in this case is a frequency-modulated signal.

The time-domain behavior of an FM phase-locked oscillation is markedly different from the time-domain behavior of an AM phase-locked oscillation. Whereas an AM phase-locked oscillation is equivalent to a pulse-modulated single-frequency signal, an FM phase-locked oscillation is equivalent to a signal whose frequency "swings" back and forth across the oscillation band-width of the laser at a rate equal to the difference frequency between adjacent longitudinal modes. The output power of an FM phase-locked laser is thus, to a first approximation, constant in time.

Although the detailed properties of AM and FM phase-locked oscillations are quite different, they both represent "coherent" signals in the sense that, if the phase of any one component of the oscillation is known, then the phase of any other component is completely predictable. It is this fact that enables one to convert a multimode oscillation to a single-frequency oscillation, with no loss in power.

Two systems have been suggested for obtaining single-frequency output beams from multimode lasers. The first system, which uses a technique called "frequency-selective coupling," is illustrated in Figure 5-3. The reflectance

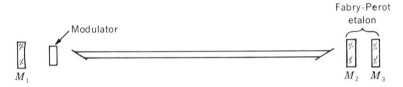

FIG. 5-3.   Frequency-selective output coupling.

of the mirrors M_1, M_2, and M_3 is chosen to be as high as possible. Mirrors M_2 and M_3 constitute a Fabry-Perot etalon which has a high transmission for one longitudinal mode and a high reflectance for the remaining longi-tudinal modes. Since (in an ideal situation) output coupling is provided for only one longitudinal mode, the output from the laser will be a single-frequency beam.

In the absence of any coupling between the modes of the laser, the above system will not work at all. All the modes except the desired mode will oscillate strongly, but the desired mode will be below threshold.

When coupling is introduced between the modes, however, the situation will be quite different. As noted above, the function of the modulator is to produce sidebands on the various longitudinal modes at the frequencies of the adjacent longitudinal modes. If the sideband power created at the frequency of the mode which has nonzero output coupling is large enough to overcome the coupling losses seen by that mode, then the mode will oscillate, and the laser will emit a single-frequency beam.

In order for the method of frequency-selective coupling to work, there is a threshold value for the amount of modulation introduced by the modulator.

Once this threshold is exceeded, all the longitudinal modes of the laser will lock in phase.

By properly adjusting the coupling for the desired mode and the modulation depth introduced by the modulator, it is possible (in an ideal situation) to obtain all the output power potentially available from a multimode phase-locked laser as a single-frequency signal. The reason for this is that power created in any longitudinal mode of the laser can be shifted in frequency by the modulator until it appears in the mode for which output coupling is provided.

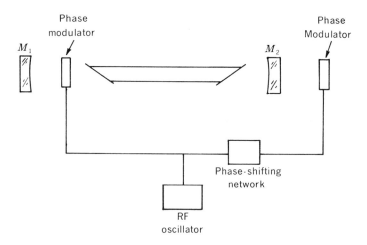

FIG. 5-4.   A "supermode" laser.

The method of frequency-selective coupling can in principle be used with either an AM or FM phase-locked laser. It is important, of course, that the Fabry-Perot etalon and the laser cavity be stabilized so that they have a common resonance frequency.

An alternate method for obtaining a single-frequency output beam from an FM phase-locked laser uses the rather poetically named "supermode" technique, illustrated in Figure 5-4. In the supermode technique, the laser is FM-modulated, and the output beam is coupled in the normal manner. The output beam is then passed through an external modulator, whose modulation depth and phase are suitably adjusted relative to those of the internal modulator so that the signal emerging from the external modulator is a single-frequency signal. If the beam emerging from the laser is a pure FM signal, then it is possible, in principle, to convert the beam to a single-frequency beam with a conversion efficiency of 100 percent.

5-3 FREQUENCY STABILIZATION OF GAS LASERS

The problem of obtaining a single-frequency output beam from a laser is closely related to the problem of stabilizing the frequency of the laser. For example, if the frequency of a short single-mode laser drifts in time, the output power of the laser will also drift in time. If the cavity length is so short that the spacing between adjacent longitudinal modes is much larger than the linewidth of the laser transition, the output power will drop to zero whenever there is no cavity resonance within the amplification bandwidth of the laser transition.

In this section, we shall consider some general problems relating to the frequency stabilization of gas lasers and shall describe some of the specific techniques that have been suggested for solving these problems.

There are two different motives for stabilizing the frequency of gas lasers. The first is the one mentioned above: it is necessary to have at least some degree of frequency stability in a single-frequency laser so that its output power will remain constant in time. The degree of stability demanded by this requirement is not particularly high. The other motivation for frequency stabilization is to construct an optical frequency standard; this, of course, places much more stringent demands on the required stability.

It is not yet clear what the eventual limits on the stability of gas lasers will be. It is clear, however, that one can fairly easily make lasers which have long-term stabilities[1] of a few parts in 10^9. Long-term stabilities of a few parts in 10^{10} have been demonstrated experimentally, and it is plausible to assume that with a real effort one might do better than this. At the current stage of gas laser technology, however, there do not appear to be any immediate applications for such stable oscillators, and comparatively little effort has been devoted to studying the phenomena which ultimately limit the stability of gas lasers.

The "gross" stability of a gas laser is, of course, determined by the requirement that the laser frequency occur within the amplification bandwidth of the laser transition. The quality factor associated with a typical visible laser transition is on the order of 10^6, so that if a laser oscillates at all, its frequency is determined to this accuracy.

Apart from the above requirement, the frequency of the laser is determined by the cavity resonance condition. It is thus important to make the laser cavity a rigid structure and to isolate it from vibration. If this is done, there

---

[1] The additional problem of absolute reproducibility is more complicated, and it is not clear what the eventual limits will be. It appears that it will always be more difficult to tune a laser to a given frequency than it will be to maintain its stability.

remain three principal factors which determine the stability (or, more properly the long-term drift) of the laser frequency:

1. The thermal expansion of the mechanical structure
2. The thermal coefficient of the refractive index of intracavity optics (windows)
3. Barometric pressure changes

The effect of the first two factors can (in principle) be eliminated by using a thermally compensated mechanical structure, and the effect of the third factor can be eliminated by keeping the atmosphere out of the laser cavity.

There is, of course, a limit on the stability that can be achieved by careful design. In practice, this limit is usually set by vibration. In order to increase the stability beyond this limit, it is necesssary to employ some type of feedback mechanism which will correct for vibrational effects (and residual deficiencies in the thermal stability). By mounting the laser mirrors on piezoelectric cells, it is possible to control the cavity length with a high degree of precision; the main problem in making a servo-stabilized laser is to obtain a suitable error signal to drive the mirrors.[2]

The basic requirements for a suitable error signal are (1) that it have a magnitude proportional to the amount of length correction required and (2) that it indicate the direction of the required length correction. There are a number of ways to obtain such an error signal. In the rest of this section we shall consider some of the schemes that have been proposed.

It is convenient to classify stabilization schemes into two categories: those which stabilize the laser frequency to that of a passive cavity, and those which stabilize the laser frequency to that of the atomic transition.

In a sense, the stabilization schemes which utilize passive cavities merely transfer the stability problem from one cavity to another. There can be considerable practical advantage in doing this: It is much easier to isolate a small passive cavity from thermal, atmospheric, and vibrational effects than it is to isolate the laser cavity itself.

There have been a wide variety of schemes proposed which utilize passive cavities for laser stabilization. One of the simplest is to send the laser beam through an ordinary Fabry-Perot etalon whose plate separation is slightly modulated at an audio frequency. The output beam from the etalon is detected by a photodetector. If the laser frequency coincides with the resonance

---

[2] One must also, of course, consider such factors as the bandwidth and stability of the servosystem.

frequency of the etalon, the output photocurrent will contain only even harmonics of the modulation frequency. By measuring the amplitude and phase of the third harmonic of the modulation frequency, an error signal can be obtained to control the cavity length of the laser.

Of the stabilization schemes which stabilize the laser frequency to that of the atomic line, the one which is currently most widely used is based on the fact that, because of the Lamb dip, the output power from a single-longitudinal-mode gas laser will have a local minimum when the frequency of oscillation occurs at the center of the atomic transition. By modulating the cavity length at an audio frequency and recovering the third harmonic of the modulation frequency from the output beam, it is possible to derive an error signal to stabilize the laser frequency on the center of the atomic transition. This scheme has the disadvantage, of course, that the output beam from the laser is frequency-modulated, but the amount of modulation needed to derive the error signal is small (~ 5 MHz), and in many applications the presence of the FM is of no consequence.

It is possible to derive an error signal to stabilize a gas laser by using an external absorption cell. The advantages obtained from using an external absorption cell rather than the laser itself are analogous to those obtained from using an external passive cavity rather than the laser cavity itself: namely, it is easier to control the discharge conditions in an external absorption cell than it is to control the discharge conditions in the laser. One way to derive an error signal from an external absorption cell is to place the cell in a magnetic field. Right- and left-handed circularly polarized laser beams which pass through the cell in the direction of the magnetic field will, in general, be differentially absorbed by the cell, because of circular dichroism introduced by Zeeman splitting of the laser transition. However, if the frequency of the incoming laser beam is at line center, the differential absorption will disappear. By using a suitable collection of polarizing optics, this effect can be used to obtain an error signal which will stabilize the laser frequency at line center.

It is also possible to obtain an error signal by putting an internal-mirror laser in a magnetic field. The circular dichroism introduced by Zeeman splitting will then favor a right- or left-handed circularly polarized mode unless the laser is tuned exactly to line center. Depending on the J values of the upper and lower energy levels of the laser transition, the right- and left-handed circularly polarized modes can be either strongly coupled or weakly coupled, in the sense described in Chapter 3. If the modes are weakly coupled, this method yields an error signal which is a very sensitive function of the displacement of the laser oscillation frequency from line center.

It is possible to stabilize the frequency of a multimode FM phase-locked laser. If a laser is FM phase-locked to a "carrier" frequency which is located precisely at line center, then (in an ideal situation) the output beam from the laser will be a pure FM signal. Such a beam will produce no power at the difference frequency between adjacent longitudinal modes when it is detected by a photodetector. (The upper sidebands will be out of phase with the lower sidebands.) On the other hand, if the carrier frequency is slightly detuned from line center, there will be "AM distortion" on the FM oscillation, which will create power at the difference frequency between adjacent longitudinal modes when the beam is detected by a photodetector. By measuring the amplitude and relative phase of this beat-frequency signal, an error signal can be obtained to stabilize the carrier of the FM oscillation on line center.

REFERENCES

1. S. E. Harris, *Appl. Optics*, **5**: 1639 (1966).

This is a good review article on the characteristics of phase-locked lasers.

2. A. D. White, *IEEE J. Quantum Electronics*, **QE-1**: 349 (1965); G. Birnbaum, *Proc. IEEE*, **55**: 1015 (1967).

These two papers review the current state of the art concerning the frequency stabilization of gas lasers.

6 OUTPUT POWER OF GAS LASERS

One of the most important properties of a gas laser is its output power.[1] In this chapter we shall consider the factors that determine this property. It is convenient to divide the discussion into two parts: in the first part of this chapter we shall consider the single-mode laser, for which an exact solution for the output power can be obtained; in the second part of this chapter we shall consider an approximate solution for the output intensity of a multimode laser.

6-1 SINGLE-MODE GAS LASERS

The fundamental equation determining the output intensity of a single-mode gas laser was derived in Chapter 3. In the present discussion, we shall confine our interest to line center, so that the equation defining the intensity of an oscillation in a single-mode gas laser [Eq. (3-38)] becomes

$$\alpha_t = \frac{g_{t0}}{\sqrt{\pi}\,[1 + (W/W_s)]^{1/2}}\, Z_i\left[i\frac{\gamma'}{\Delta\omega_D}\left(1 + \frac{W}{W_s}\right)^{1/2}\right] \tag{6-1}$$

It is convenient to rewrite this equation in terms of the unsaturated temporal gain coefficient at line center:

$$g'_{t0} = \frac{g_{t0}}{\sqrt{\pi}}\, Z_i\left(i\frac{\gamma'}{\Delta\omega_D}\right) \tag{6-2}$$

[1] The output power of a laser is equal to the output intensity times the cross-sectional area of the beam.

113

We then have

$$\frac{g_{t0}'}{\alpha_t} = X = \left(1 + \frac{W}{W_s}\right)^{\frac{1}{2}} \frac{Z_i[i(\gamma'/\Delta\omega_D)]}{Z_i\{i(\gamma'/\Delta\omega_D)[1 + (W/W_s)]^{\frac{1}{2}}\}} \qquad (6\text{-}3)$$

where X is the excitation parameter defined in Chapter 3. The excitation parameter can be expressed in terms of the unsaturated gain per pass at line center, G_0', for a wave propagating back and forth between the laser mirrors. We have

$$G_0' = \frac{L}{c} g_{t0}' \qquad (6\text{-}4)$$

The excitation parameter then becomes

$$X = \frac{G_0'}{1 - r} \qquad (6\text{-}5)$$

where r is the reflectance of the laser mirrors. If the mirrors have transmittance t and loss[2] a, then

$$1 - r = a + t$$

so that

$$X = \frac{G_0'}{a + t} \qquad (6\text{-}7)$$

The output intensity of a single-mode laser is determined by the requirement that the intracavity intensity stabilize at a level such that Eq. (6-3) is satisfied. The output intensity is then

$$W_{\text{out}} = tW \qquad (6\text{-}8)$$

Unfortunately, Eq. (6-3) is an "implicit" solution for the intracavity intensity. In general, it is not possible to invert the equation, and solutions must be obtained graphically. However, if the laser transition is inhomogeneous, then the ratio of the plasma dispersion functions in Eq. (6-3) is unity, and we find a solution

$$W = W_s(X^2 - 1) \qquad (6\text{-}9)$$

The output intensity is then conveniently expressed in normalized form by

$$\frac{W_{\text{out}}}{a} = \frac{tW}{a} = \frac{t}{a} W_s\left[\frac{(G_0'/a)^2}{(1 + t/a)^2} - 1\right] \qquad (6\text{-}10)$$

---

[2] We use the general term "loss" to describe the effects of absorption, scattering, and diffraction.

If the laser transition is homogeneous, then we can use Eq. (2-102) to show that

$$W = W_s(X - 1) \qquad (6-11)$$

so that the output intensity can be written in normalized form as

$$\frac{W_{out}}{a} = \frac{t}{a} W = \frac{t}{a} W_s \left\{ \frac{G_0'/a}{[1 + (t/a)]} - 1 \right\} \qquad (6-12)$$

For a fixed gain and loss, the output intensity is a function of the mirror transmittance t. The optimum value of the transmittance (that is, the value of the transmittance which maximizes the output intensity) is determined by the requirement that

$$\left. \frac{\partial W_{out}}{\partial t} \right|_{t=t_{opt}} = 0 \qquad (6-13)$$

For a homogeneous line, the optimum transmittance is

$$\frac{t_{opt}}{a} = \sqrt{\frac{G_0'}{a}} - 1 \qquad (6-14)$$

For an inhomogeneous line, the use of Eq. (6-10) in (6-13) leads to an implicit solution for the optimum transmittance:

$$\frac{[1 + (t_{opt}/a)]^3}{1 - (t_{opt}/a)} = \left[\frac{G_0'}{a} \right]^2 \qquad (6-15)$$

The maximum output intensity from the laser can be found by inserting these equations in Eqs. (6-12) and (6-10). For a homogeneous line we find

$$\left(\frac{W_{out}}{a} \right)_{max} = W_s \left(\sqrt{\frac{G_0'}{a}} - 1 \right)^2 \qquad (6-16)$$

and for an inhomogeneous line we find an implicit solution:

$$\left(\frac{W_{out}}{a} \right)_{max} = 2W_s \left[\frac{(t_{opt}/a)^2}{1 - (t_{opt}/a)} \right] \qquad (6-17)$$

Unfortunately, most gas-laser transitions cannot be considered either homogeneous or inhomogeneous. The intermediate broadening situation must be treated numerically or graphically by using Eq. (6-3). In Figure 6-1 is shown the solution for the optimum transmittance/loss versus gain/loss for a transition having a broadening parameter $\eta = .08$. Also shown in this

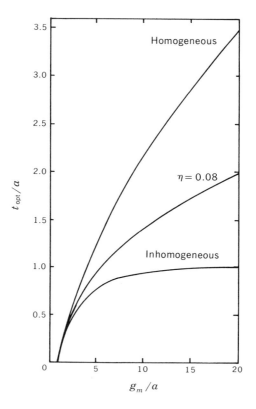

FIG. 6-1.   Optimum output coupling for a laser.

figure are the solutions (6-14) and (6-15) for homogeneous and inhomogeneous lines.

In Figure 6-2 is shown the solution for the maximum output intensity/loss versus gain/loss for a laser transition having a broadening parameter $\eta = .08$, together with the solutions (6-16) and (6-17) for homogeneous and inhomogeneous lines.

It is important to realize the role of cavity loss in determining the output intensity of a gas laser. Loss and gain do not enter the equations for the output intensity in the same way; an increase in loss will reduce the output intensity more than an equal increase in gain will enhance it, even for a homogeneously broadened laser transition.

The discussion in this section has shown that the output intensity of a laser increases as the gain of the laser increases. Thus, for example, as the length of a laser is increased, the output intensity increases (assuming, of course, that the gain coefficient is held constant). However, it does not follow

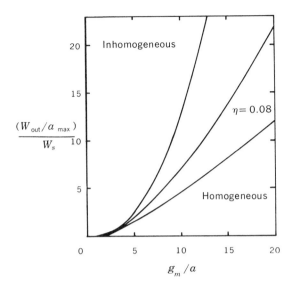

FIG. 6-2.   Output intensity of a laser.

from this discussion that lasers having large gain coefficients have correspond-
ingly high output intensities. The reason for this apparent paradox can be
seen by considering the relation of the gain coefficient to the saturation
parameter. Using Eqs. (2-66) and (2-84), we have that

$$W_s = \frac{\gamma_a \gamma_b \hbar^2 \epsilon_0 c}{2\mu^2} \tag{6-18}$$

and

$$G'_0 = \frac{\sqrt{\pi}\ \omega\mu^2 \mathcal{I}_0 L}{c\epsilon_0 \hbar\, \Delta\omega_D} \tag{6-19}$$

In a typical (good) laser, the decay from the lower laser state will be rapid
compared with the decay from the upper state. We then have that $\gamma_b \gg \gamma_a$,
so that we can write $\mathcal{I}_0$ as

$$\mathcal{I}_0 \approx \frac{\Lambda_a}{\gamma_a} \tag{6-20}$$

The intracavity intensity in a homogeneously broadened laser operating well
above threshold is given approximately by [see Eq. (6-11)]

$$W = W_s \frac{G'_0}{a + t} \tag{6-21}$$

Using Eqs. (6-19) through (6-21), we find that

$$W = \frac{\sqrt{\pi}\, \gamma_b L\hbar\omega}{2\,\Delta\omega_D(a + t)}\, \Lambda_a \tag{6-22}$$

The factor $\sqrt{\pi}\, \gamma_b/2\,\Delta\omega_D$ is of the order of unity. If we neglect this factor, we obtain for the intracavity intensity

$$W = \frac{L\hbar\omega}{a + t}\, \Lambda_a \tag{6-23}$$

Thus the intracavity intensity (and hence the output intensity) is independent of the gain coefficient and depends only on the excitation rate to the upper laser level.

The above example illustrates a typical difficulty encountered in attempting to predict the output intensity of a gas laser: the problem is complicated by the multiplicity of factors involved. It is important, as the above example clearly shows, to always keep in mind which factors are constant and which are variable.

6-2 MULTIMODE GAS LASERS

The problem of predicting the output intensity of a multimode gas laser is considerably more difficult than it is for a single-mode gas laser. Not only are there several modes to consider, but as was shown in Chapter 3, there are, in general, amplitude- and frequency-modulation effects between the various modes.

The problem of predicting the output intensity of a multimode helium-neon laser has been considered by a number of investigators. Although the method of approach used in various studies is different, the essential conclusion of all is the same: the output intensity of a multimode helium-neon laser can be predicted by assuming that the total intensity of all the modes saturates the laser transition as though it were homogeneously broadened. In this approximation, the total intracavity intensity of a multimode gas laser is given by an equation analogous to Eq. (6-11):

$$W = W_0(X - 1) \tag{6-24}$$

where W_0 is an "effective" saturation parameter. For a multimode helium-neon laser, the value of W_0 is equal to approximately 30 W/cm^2.

It is not at this time definitively established that Eq. (6-24) can be used for all multimode laser systems; in fact, some experimental evidence seems to indicate that it is not so good an approximation for ion-laser transitions as it is for helium-neon transitions. Nevertheless, it can be derived by using general qualitative arguments concerning hole-burning effects, and we shall assume that Eq. (6-24) gives an adequate approximation for the intracavity intensity of all multimode gas lasers.

Since a multimode laser behaves as though the laser transition were homogeneously broadened, the optimum transmittance for the laser mirrors is given by Eq. (6-14). The output intensity is determined by an equation like (6-16), except that for a multimode laser the effective saturation parameter W_0 must be used.

To demonstrate the use of Eq. (6-24), it is worth calculating the output power of a typical helium-neon laser. To begin, we may note that the gain coefficient for the helium-neon 6328-Å laser transition has been experimentally measured to be

$$g_l = \frac{3 \times 10^{-4}}{d} \tag{6-25}$$

where d is the diameter of the plasma tube.

The output beam from most helium-neon lasers is obtained from one end of the laser; in such lasers it is desirable to use a "backup" mirror (that is, the mirror at the opposite end of the laser) having as high a reflectance as possible. In calculating the output power of such lasers, it is most convenient to express the excitation parameter in terms of round-trip gains and losses. We thus have

$$X = \frac{2g_l L}{a + t} = \frac{6 \times 10^{-4} L/d}{a + t} \tag{6-26}$$

where t is the output-mirror transmittance, and a is the sum of:

1. The transmittance, scatter, and absorption of the backup mirror
2. Four times the loss obtained in passing through a Brewster window
3. The absorption and scatter in the output mirror
4. The diffraction loss for the laser mode

The output intensity of the laser is thus [see Eq. (6-24)]

$$W_{\text{out}} = tW_0 \left[\frac{6 \times 10^{-4} L/d}{a + t} - 1 \right] \tag{6-27}$$

The output power of the laser is equal to the above times the cross-sectional area of the output beam. For lasers using long-radius cavities running in the

TEM$_{00}$ transverse mode, the effective cross-sectional area of the output beam
has been found (experimentally) to be approximately $\frac{1}{5}$ the cross-sectional
area of the plasma-tube bore. We thus have

$$P_{\text{out}} = tW_0\left(\frac{\pi d^2}{4}\right)\left(\frac{1}{5}\right)\left[\frac{6 \times 10^{-4}L/d}{a + t} - 1\right] \qquad \text{watts} \qquad (6\text{-}28)$$

or

$$P_{\text{out}} = 4700td^2\left[\frac{6 \times 10^{-4}L/d}{a + t} - 1\right] \qquad \text{milliwatts} \qquad (6\text{-}29)$$

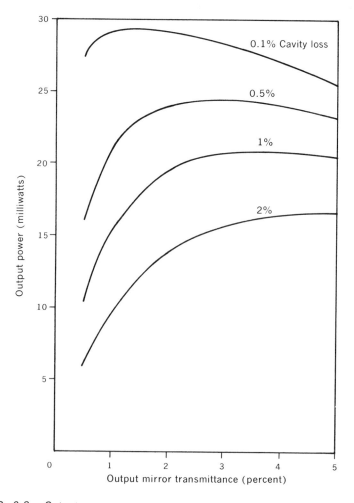

FIG. 6-3.   Output power versus output coupling for a helium-neon laser.

Figures 6-3 and 6-4 show graphs of Eq. (6-29) for a specific helium-neon laser having a discharge length of 65 cm and a plasma-tube-bore diameter of 1.7 mm. In Figure 6-3, the output power is plotted versus output-mirror transmittance for various values of intracavity loss. In Figure 6-4, the output power is plotted versus intracavity loss for various values of the output-mirror transmittance. These graphs are in good agreement with experimental data.

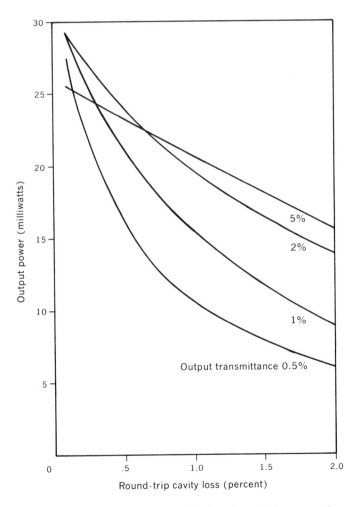

FIG. 6-4.   Output power versus cavity loss for a helium-neon laser.

REFERENCES

1. W. W. Rigrod, *J. Appl. Phys.*, **34**: 2602 (1963); A. D. White, E. I. Gordon, and J. D. Rigden, *Appl. Phys. Letters*, **2**: 91 (1963); P. W. Smith, *IEEE J. Quantum Electronics*, **QE-2**: 62 (1966).

These three papers discuss the output power of gas lasers. Smith's paper is the only one that adequately treats the single-mode laser, although all of them obtain similar results for multimode lasers.

7 CONSTRUCTION OF GAS LASERS

The construction of gas lasers is one of the most interesting and challenging problems in experimental physics, because a wide variety of different disciplines must be combined to produce the final result. Materials technology, vacuum technology, electrical design, mechanical design, and optical design must all be coordinated to produce a gas laser.

In this chapter, we shall attempt to describe some of the aspects of the above disciplines that are applicable to gas-laser technology. It would be impossible, in a work of this size, to give a complete treatment of the subject. We have, however, tried to describe the salient aspects of gas-laser construction, as well as to include some detailed descriptions of experimental techniques that have not been described in the literature.

7–1 GAS-LASER PLASMA TUBES

The plasma tube is the heart of the gas laser and is usually the most expensive and failure-prone component of the system. Although the art of confining gas discharges in vacuum-tight envelopes has had a long and successful history (for example, in neon signs, mercury arcs, and gas rectifiers) the stringent requirements of the gas laser have made the simple extrapolation of established gas-discharge-tube design difficult. The technology involves at least two new basic requirements which are still in a state of evolution. The first is the termination of both ends of a confined long positive column by a substantially loss-free optical system. The second is the capability of sustaining a relatively low-pressure discharge for long periods of time without cleaning up the gas or developing impurities which will destroy the gas amplifier or degrade the optics.

Plasma-tube design criteria can be divided into two general classes according to the plasma properties: (1) glow-discharge systems such as the helium-neon and (2) arc-discharge systems such as the argon-ion. The mercury-ion system, which is unusual in that laser action can be obtained in a hollow-cathode discharge, will therefore be treated as a special case.

The modest power requirements of the glow-discharge lasers do not impose any stringent requirements for materials resistant to thermal shock, since no special cooling of the capillary is required. For this reason, the easily worked borosilicate glasses are almost always used when the glow discharge is excited by direct current. For radio-frequency-excited tubes, fused silica is generally used to minimize wall losses. The most important glow-discharge laser system is the visible helium-neon at 6328 Å, and the plasma-tube geometry has been studied in detail to yield optimum performance.

The most useful plasma-tube configurations appear to be those which yield uniphase optical output by combining long-radius cavity structures with narrow bores. The effect of the competing infrared transition at 3.39 μ is particularly severe for these tubes,[1] and it is necessary to use special techniques to suppress the infrared oscillation.

Three approaches have been used: wavelength selection in the optical cavity, a methane absorbing cell in the optical cavity, and Zeeman broadening of the spectral lines by inhomogeneous magnetic fields along the plasma tube. The first two are quite effective until the bore length is long enough so that the amplification of 3.39-μ radiation is large enough to deplete appreciably

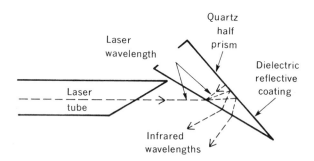

FIG. 7-1.   Infrared suppression by an intracavity prism.

[1] The 3.39-μ and 6328-Å laser transitions share a common upper level, and oscillation at 3.39 μ will reduce the output power on the 6328-Å transition.

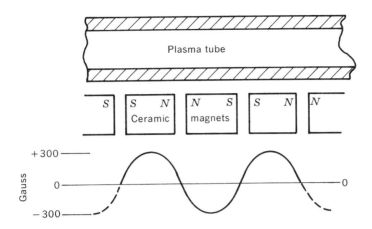

FIG. 7-2. Infrared suppression by inhomogeneous broadening of 3.39-μ transition.

the population of the upper laser state. At this point a combination of both cavity and magnet suppression is needed. Figure 7-1 illustrates the use of a half-prism cut so that 6328-Å light entering the prism at Brewster's angle will be retroreflected from the back-surface coating while rejecting the unwanted infrared.

Infrared suppression can also be accomplished by placing small ceramic magnets along the plasma tube as shown in Figure 7-2. The mechanism of this method is the Zeeman splitting of the 6328-Å and 3.39-μ transitions. Both lines are equally broadened, but since the Doppler width of the 6328-Å line is considerably larger, the gain is not appreciably affected when weak inhomogeneous fields are used. A uniform field is much less effective because it splits the infrared transition into only two components, each having significant gain.

The detailed geometry of helium-neon plasma tubes is of no special significance (with the exception, of course, of the length and diameter of the active region). It is generally most convenient to place the cathode and anode in side appendages, although a number of coaxial designs have proved successful.

With standard glass-cutting equipment, the ends of the tube are cut off at the complement of Brewster's angle. Errors of a fraction of a degree are generally tolerable for these cuts. The Brewster windows themselves are most commonly fastened to the plasma tube with an epoxy cement, such as Hysol 1-C or Varian Torr-Seal.

Getters are often placed in plasma tubes to maintain the purity of the gas. The most common sort are the conventional barium getters used in electron tubes.

Laser action has been observed in the gaseous ions of many elements, but only the noble gases (particularly argon and krypton) have received extensive study and development to the present. Most of the engineering problems yet to be solved pertain to the plasma tube, which must confine a very hot gas for an appreciable period of time to be useful. The first successful cw gas-ion-laser plasma tubes were constructed of water-cooled fused silica, and this material continues to dominate experimental ion laser construction because of the ease with which it may be fabricated. The main limitations derive from the very low thermal conductivity, which sets an upper limit on the power input per unit area of the capillary bore, particularly at the cathode end of dc-arc tubes, where an anomalously high gas temperature is encountered. In fact, most of the plasma-tube failures result from erosion of the cathode throat. A number of investigators have studied other materials and construction techniques in a search for an engineering solution to this problem.

One of the first approaches was the use of a more refractory material for plasma-tube construction. It is worth reviewing some of the earlier experience gained in this effort as a background for future work.

The oxide ceramics—alumina, beryllia, and magnesia—are all superior to fused silica in their resistance to devitrification at high temperatures, but this advantage is countered to some extent by their poor thermal-shock resistance and by fabrication problems involving the ceramics themselves. It was soon discovered that long, straight precision-bore capillaries were not easy to make in oxide ceramics and were often strained in manufacture. The net effect of such strain would be a catastrophic rupture of the bore when the first arc was struck. Assuming that a strain-free bore was selected, the problem of making a vacuum-tight transition from ceramic to glass to complete the plasma-tube structure usually involved a large thermal gradient at the throat seal, where maximum heat transfer was needed. This problem in thermal and vacuum topology was undoubtedly responsible for the failure of many ingenious designs. However, the oxide-ceramic approach, especially with beryllia, is sufficiently promising that a satisfactory structure is likely to evolve.

One material that looked particularly promising at the outset was boron nitride. The physical properties of the pure material are ideal: high thermal conductivity and shock resistance; easily machined to high tolerances, with good electrical insulation. However, it cannot be bonded to other materials in vacuum-tight transitions except by mechanical compression seals. If this where the only disadvantage, boron nitride would indeed be very attractive, but experimental plasma tubes of this material have failed because of the continuous evolution of impurity gases such as oxygen and the subsequent rapid erosion of the capillary wall. It would appear that the boric oxide binder used in the manufacture decomposes in the presence of the hot plasma, leaving a porous boron nitride matrix with a degraded thermal conductivity. The result is a runaway capillary failure after a few hours of operation. It is possible that the recent availability of pyrolitic boron nitride containing no binder material may alleviate this serious limitation and permit a reevaluation of this attractive substance for plasma confinement.

A number of laboratories have investigated the possibility of using segmented metal bores for plasma-confining capillaries. The design is based on the fact that a coaxial stack of metal disks insulated from each other will not provide an alternate path for the discharge, provided that the arc drop in volts per disk thickness is less than the work function to extract electrons from the metal. It is clear that metals can provide an ideal heat sink because of good thermal conductivity and freedom from thermal shock, but the presence of ions in the discharge still gives rise to bore erosion by the sputtering process, and again the cathode throat is most rapidly attacked at the glow-to-arc transition region. Most of these structures have used radiation cooling of the metal disks as a means of dissipating the plasma heat, which aggravates the sputtering problem because of the high temperatures that the disks must reach to radiate effectively. The disk material is usually a refractory metal such as tungsten or molybdenum, and one is faced with the secondary problem that oxide cathode emission can be seriously degraded by traces of these metals on the surface.

Segmented graphite bores have been tried with varying degrees of success. The high thermal emissivity and high sputtering potential of graphite are definitely attractive, but it would appear that the processing recipe for reproducible plasma tubes is very critical to avoiding the gas storage and release which seems responsible for some of the graphite dust found distributed in these plasma tubes after a period of operation.

We may summarize the preceding discussion on the state of the art for cw gas-ion plasma tubes by saying that the technology for tubes other than fused-silica ones is still evolving, and it appears that a long and expensive development program is likely. We shall therefore confine ourselves to fabrication of fused-silica tubes in our recipe for experimental gas-ion lasers. Many workers have noticed a wide variation in the behavior of this material in the presence of a hot plasma, and perhaps some of the idiosyncrasies may be explained by reviewing the manufacturing process.

Fused silica is made by melting quartz sand in an electric furnace. The crystalline particles will begin to fuse together at about 1400°C and will become a molasses-like viscous mass at about 1700°C. The transition from crystalline quartz to vitreous fused silica involves a volume expansion of about 17 percent, which then undergoes a slight shrinkage on cooling to room temperature. The most desirable physical properties are those of clear transparent billets, which are obtained by vacuum outgassing of the highly viscous melt. These are then extruded or shaped by carbon mandrels to the desired physical form.

In service, fused silica will undergo devitrification starting at about 1100°C. The material slowly turns white and granular, weakens, and loses its very low coefficient of expansion. The most common impurity in natural quartz is iron, which begins to color fused silica visibly at about 10 parts per million, and probably accounts for some of the variations observed in plasma-tube processing and performance.

A procedure that has provided plasma capillaries of acceptable lifetime begins with a selection of clear, precision-bore fused silica, free from bubbles and striae. The wall thickness is chosen so that the inner wall does not reach the devitrification temperature for a given power per unit area of input.

The tube is then vacuum-shrunk to the desired bore size on a polished tungsten mandrel in a glass lathe. The shrinkage is nominally 10 percent of the original bore diameter, and the tungsten mandrel should be held taut between chucks to ensure straightness. This procedure ensures that the longitudinal marks left in the tubing by the original extrusion process will not be the source of incipient capillary cracking under high thermal gradients. After cooling and removal of the mandrel, the capillary is washed and checked with a ×50 stereo microscope, using the capillary as a light pipe. Any capillaries with scratches or aberrations are rejected for reworking. Except for very short bores, the capillary must be provided with a bellows to allow for differential expansion. A typical design is shown in Figure 7-3. The optimum design of the capillary throat has been the subject of considerable speculation because of the anomalously high plasma temperatures encountered at the glow-to-arc transition. However, no particular shape that has been tested, such as the straight taper or exponential horn, has shown any magic in suppressing the excessive bore erosion in this region.

The bore and water jacket are usually constructed as a unit and can be used for either the induction ring discharge or the dc-arc tubes. Some of the early dc-arc tube designs provided coaxial cathodes and anodes on the bore axis. Although this yields a compact design, these structures tend to be a source of window contamination through evaporation or sputtering processes, and the placing of the electrodes in side-arm tubes now seems to be preferred.

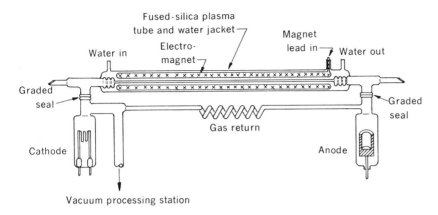

FIG. 7-3.   A direct-current-excited cw gas-ion laser tube.

In either case (dc or rf), however, it is important to keep the windows free of any contact with the glowing plasma.

The capillary section of the rf-excited ring discharge tubes is identical to those of the dc arcs, but the slight modification to complete the gas ring offers a considerable simplification of the complete plasma tube; that is, graded seals are eliminated along with the cathode and anode. The complete absence of metal structures and sensitive cathode surfaces makes the tube not only very tolerant of impurities but also capable of cw laser action with highly

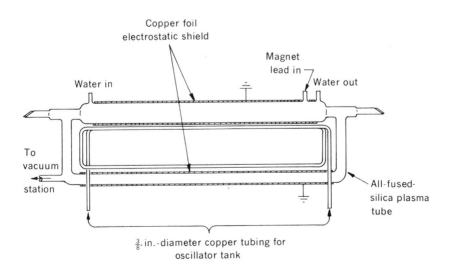

FIG. 7-4.   A radio-frequency-excited cw gas-ion laser plasma tube.

reactive gases such as chlorine. Figure 7-4 shows a typical rf-excited ion laser tube.

The mercury ion is unusual in that it provides high gain with the largest aperture of any visible laser. Where pulsed operation is not objectionable, this laser is very easily fabricated to give long and reliable performance.

Two configurations of this laser have been developed which have proved useful: (1) the pulsed positive-column arc discharge and (2) the follow cathode. The former is the simplest form, and its fabrication can be easily accomplished with modest facilities. The plasma-tube geometry is shown in Figure 7-5.

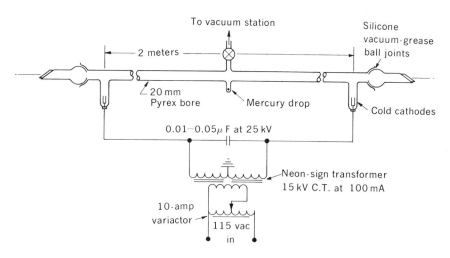

FIG. 7-5. A "positive-column" mercury-ion laser tube. (*Note:* Freeze mercury with dry-ice cold trap when processing; operate at 30 to 40°C with stopcock closed.)

For a bore diameter of 20 mm and a length of 2 m, the gain at the 5677-Å transition will approach 100 percent with natural mercury and the simple pulser shown. The plasma tube is most easily fabricated from Pyrex glass with ball-joint ends, using ordinary neon-sign cold cathodes.

The mercury-ion hollow-cathode laser is perhaps the more useful configuration but is much more complex. It has the advantage of very reproducible pulse behavior, with the laser output occurring during the pulse rather than in the afterglow. The gains with isotopic mercury 202 are 5 to 10 dB/m in the hollow-cathode structure shown in Figure 7-6. These structures have been successfully built up to 2 in. in diameter with laser action over the full aperture. The only visible line obtained is at 6150 Å. The Doppler width corresponds to mercury at room temperature, and this narrow line is potentially useful as a wavelength standard.

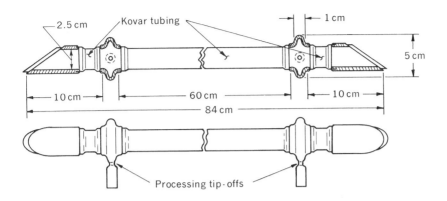

FIG. 7-6.   A "hollow-cathode" mercury-ion laser tube.

The plasma tube is constructed of thin-wall Kovar tubing and Kovar-sealing glass. The metal-tubing ends are flared slightly to ensure full aperture after the glassing operation. To ensure a homogeneous plasma distribution, it is important that no sharp points or radii in the metal structure be exposed to the discharge. The glassing operation is carried out on a graphite mandrel in a lathe in order to keep the structure strictly coaxial. A thorough cleaning operation is subsequently required to remove the tenacious Kovar metal oxides before window sealing and processing.

The most important aspect of plasma-tube assembly is the development of a procedure which will yield a minimum contamination of the Brewster windows. These relatively cool parts of the plasma tend to collect any condensable impurities or sputtered metal vapors from the electrodes. The most desirable designs place the electrodes and getters well away from the windows and permit a processing technique that allows the use of temporary seals at the plasma tube ends. For experimental plasma tubes that stay on the vacuum station, the use of Brewster windows or internal mirrors attached to ball joints has proved to be a versatile procedure for easily changing and adjusting the optical system.

A rather generalized sequence for plasma-tube assembly might follow this recipe: The capillary is selected for uniform bore, wall thickness, and straightness. Side terminations are blown, and ends are cut and polished. This structure is carefully cleaned with a 5 percent HF and distilled-water solution, followed by a distilled-water rinse and drying in a warm oven. Cathode and anode assemblies are glassed on through a drying tube, and the structure leak is checked with a forepump vacuum and a tesla coil. The bore is then inspected for dust particles by using it as light pipe from a microscope illuminator. The complete plasma tube is then glassed to the vacuum station and processed with dummy optics where possible. The final optical components are placed on the tube when clean operation of the plasma discharge is obtained. Air can be prevented from making contact with processed plasma tubes by keeping a slight overpressure of dry argon or nitrogen in the vacuum manifold when changing the optics.

7–2 CATHODES FOR PLASMA TUBES

Gas-laser cathodes are subjected to working environments that are considerably more abusive than their high-vacuum counterparts and, as would be expected, are still undergoing development toward providing long, reliable life. The emission requirements cover two extremes: the fractional-ampere region for glow discharges and the multiampere region required for the gas-ion lasers. The usual difficulties encountered with gas-laser cathodes include: excessive sputtering, evaporation, reactivity with non-noble gases, and cleanup of the gas fill due to any of these processes. Most of these problems are greatly aggravated by the low gas pressures required for optimum laser output.

Both hot and cold cathodes have been successfully used with glow-discharge plasma tubes. Cold cathodes have advantages of economy, ruggedness, and simplicity, provided that gas cleanup rates can be kept to acceptable levels. Three types of cold emitters have been studied and used in gas lasers: oxide-coated metal hollow cathodes of the type commonly used in neon signs, cylinders of sputter-resistant metals such as aluminum, and mercury-vapor-buffered cathode structures employing gas cataphoresis.

Oxide-coated cold cathodes, as obtained from sign manufacturers, are intended for use with noble-gas mixtures at pressures of 6 to 10 torr and, when properly processed, exhibit tube lifetimes of at least 10,000 hr. The basic cathode is available in a variety of glass types. For laser work, Nonex is the most useful. The cathodes are internally coated with a suspension of barium, strontium, and calcium carbonates in a nitrocellulose binder.

A number of metals and alloys—notably aluminum, magnesium, and tantalum—exhibit exceptionally low sputtering rates when used as cold cathodes in noble-gas glow discharges. It appears that the low sputtering rate results from the formation of a refractory tenacious oxide layer on the metal surface, which is highly resistant to erosion by ion bombardment. The emission mechanism is believed to arise from electron tunneling through the thin oxide layer, because of the high electric field gradient generated by positive ions striking the cathode surface.

An interesting application of gas cataphoresis has been used to yield exceptionally long cold-cathode life in the helium-neon laser. A small drop of mercury in the cathode envelope provides an inexhaustible reservoir of vapor that is trapped at the cathode end of the glow discharge by the strong cataphoresis of mercury vapor in the highly mobile helium and neon as long as the discharge is on. The lower ionization potential of mercury permits only neutral helium and neon in the cathode area, with a corresponding sharp reduction of cathode sputtering and rare-gas cleanup rates. The principal objection to this scheme is the slow diffusion of mercury throughout the plasma tube when the discharge is off, as well as the long time taken to pump the mercury vapor back to the cathode after turn-on.

The hot-cathode structures used in gas-ion lasers have been mainly derived from their high-current gas rectifier or thyration counterparts, and a number of manufacturers have made available unprocessed cathode structures ready for sealing onto plasma tubes. Although these cathodes have exhibited long reliable life in the gas-filled tubes for which they were originally designed and have proved useful in glow-discharge tubes, their useful lifetime in gas-ion laser service suffers severely because of discharge contaminants and the low gas-filling pressures required. Some improvement can be obtained by operating at emission currents considerably below the manufacturers rating and by removing the metal heat shield surrounding the emitter. This latter modification is made to keep the cathode surface free of sputtered metal produced by ion bombardment. It is important to readjust the heater power in order to maintain the proper cathode temperature when the heat shield is removed. Although the general fabrication recipe for hot-oxide thermionic emitters is well known, each manufacturer has developed a precise fabricating and processing technique based on experience. For this reason it is preferable to purchase prefabricated cathodes and follow the activation instructions rather than to attempt to duplicate the commercial product. For those who wish to experiment with their own cathodes, an attractive alternative which has not yet appeared commercially is the rare-earth hexaboride emitter.

These last-named cathodes offer potentially a number of attractive and unique properties: they are unaffected by water or air, are resistant to ion bombardment, and are efficient emitters with low evaporation rates. Because of its very high Richardson constant, the most efficient emitter of the group is lathanum hexaboride.

The very physical properties that make the compound an attractive cathode material are, unfortunately, the properties which make fabrication difficult. The extreme reactivity of boron limits the choice of heater substrate to graphite or rhenium. Since boron does not react with graphite and reacts only at elevated temperatures with rhenium, the coating cannot be bonded to the substrate and must be applied as a mechanical adhesion to porous surfaces or

mesh. This fabrication problem has yet to be solved to the production tolerances required by high-vacuum electron tubes, but cathodes for gas-discharge
plasma tubes require little control of mechanical dimensions, and it appears
that these cathodes may be attractive for use in gas-ion laser tubes.

7–3 VACUUM PROCESSING OF PLASMA TUBES

The vacuum processing of gas-laser plasma tubes is essentially one of technique in removing both absorbed and adsorbed impurity gases from the plasma-
tube structure prior to refilling with known constituents. Experience has
shown that gas-laser performance is not seriously affected by the presence
of impurity gases up to at least 10 ppm, or approximately a partial pressure
of 10^{-5} torr for most lasers. Clearly then, a vacuum system capable of
a modest 10^{-6} torr is quite adequate if a successful plasma-tube cleaning
recipe is followed. It is also worth noting that the pumping speed of a vacuum
system, as far as the plasma tube is concerned, is basically limited by the small
aperture of the plasma-tube tip-off constriction, and large high-speed pumps
do not significantly contribute to a reduction in processing time.

Since most gas lasers use (nonreactive) noble gases, either as fillings, or
buffers, a satisfactory pumping system is also one of the most common and
consists of a mechanical forepump and an oil diffusion pump, followed by
one or more cold traps.

Gas-laser vacuum systems must have means for accurate measurement of
gas pressures ranging from 10^{-3} torr to perhaps as high as 100 torr, with
emphasis on high absolute accuracy in the region of 0.5 to 5 torr. Accurate
knowledge of the high-vacuum pressure is not essential, except to check
that the system is pumped down to 10^{-6} torr or better. In this region any
of the standard ion gauges are quite satisfactory, but these become unreliable
in the gas-laser pressure ranges. Most of the trouble stems from the gauge-
calibration dependence on the particular gas species involved, and although
a continuously reading ion or thermocouple gauge is excellent for relative
pressure changes, the calibration should be constantly checked against an
absolute gauge that can be valved into the system at any time.

The absolute gauges that have proved most useful are the mercury McLeod,
the oil manometer, and the mechanical diaphragm. The last-named is useful
as a general system-pressure check and can be quite accurate above several
torr. From several torr down to about 0.1 torr, the oil manometer is excellent
and reads continuously.

Manometers constructed using silicon oils can provide high continuous-
reading accuracy in the range of pressures used in gas-discharge lasers.

For Dow Corning 704, the density is 1.07. The gauge constant will be 12.7 mm per torr. With care, the meniscus can be read to a fraction of a millimeter to yield an absolute accuracy of ± 2 percent over the range 2 to 4 torr that is generally used in the helium-neon laser. Below 1 torr, the McLeod gauge is effective and can be read to high accuracy on an intermittent basis. It is essential that mercury and oil gauges be cold trapped to prevent diffusion of unwanted vapors from the gauge fluids.

The scope of gas-laser research has rapidly expanded to include the elements of a good part of the periodic table in the form of vapors or mixtures thereof. Generally speaking, the noble gases are handled most easily, and the reactive gases are the most difficult. Metal vapors pose a special problem because of the tight control needed on thermal gradients and because of the reactivity of many metal vapors with plasma-tube materials.

It is important that the basic-working-vacuum manifold be well isolated by cold traps in order to prevent contamination by persistent condensable vapors, such as mercury and sulfur.

A versatile vacuum processing station for experimental gas lasers is shown in Figure 7-7. The choice of borosilicate glass for the working manifold is made for a number of reasons: it is easy and quick to fabricate; leaks are easy to detect; changes or additions can be rapidly made; the system is easily outgassed by running low-pressure discharges through the manifold; and electrical isolation of the experimental plasma tube to ground is seldom a problem, especially for pulsed plasmas.

A new vacuum system invariably goes through a shakedown period before it is useful for vacuum research. Residual water vapor is the most persistent contaminant and is derived from new pump oils, gauge fluids, and the glass walls. Pumps should be run for about 24 hr to dry them out, followed by heating the glasswork wherever possible. Running a discharge through the manifold with dry nitrogen or argon at about 0.1 torr is a very effective way of speeding up the wall-cleaning process and is also a useful way to hunt for leaks. While the discharge is on, a drop of acetone can be applied to suspected areas. If a leak is present, a sudden change in discharge color will act as an indicator. This technique is particularly useful at glass-to-metal seals, where the tesla coil is ineffective. Once a system has been dried out, modifications or additions to the system should be made by letting the system up to atmospheric pressure with dry nitrogen or argon to prevent re-contamination. New glasswork should then be added by blowing through a calcium sulfate drying tube.

All the noble gases are available in 1-liter Pyrex flasks near atmospheric pressure and require special handling to assure that the initial impurities

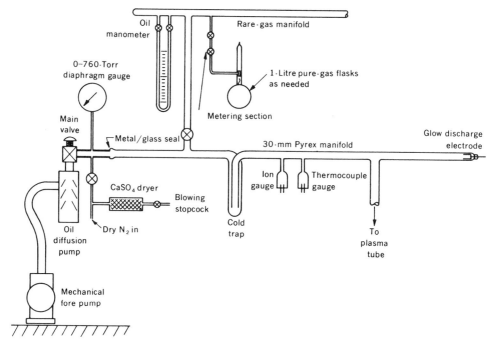

FIG. 7-7.   A vacuum system for gas-laser research.

(usually a few parts per million) are not increased during use. These gases can also be obtained premixed by the supplier, and the standard helium-neon laser ratios are now common. To introduce these gases into the manifold, a fragile glass seal must be broken under vacuum, with a double-stopcock or metal-valve metering section then regulating the flow.

The following vacuum processing recipe deals specifically with the helium-neon laser plasma tube using an oxide-coated cold cathode, although other glow-discharge tubes will follow substantially the same technique for permanently sealed-off devices.

For assemblies with epoxy-sealed optics, the tube is baked in a vacuum oven for 48 hr at a temperature of 75°C before sealing onto the vacuum station. Be sure to flame-anneal any reworked glass after seal-on and tip-off. Pump down hard (10^{-6} torr or better) and check for leaks with helium leak detector. The cathode is then ready for processsing. Figure 7-8 shows a processing supply suitable for processing oxide-coated cold cathodes. The system is then filled with tank oxygen to a pressure of about 1 to 2 torr, and a current of about 0.2 A is passed through the manifold anode to the plasma-tube cathode. Note that the processing discharge does not go through the

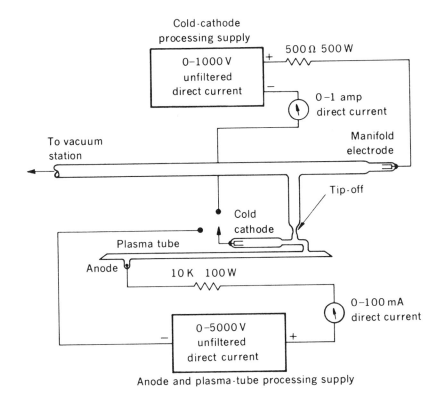

FIG. 7-8. A typical cold-cathode processing station.
(*Note:* Avoid overheating during processing.)

plasma-tube capillary. This discharge current will decompose the organic binder and yield copious amounts of hydrocarbons. As the gas accumulates, it is carefully valved out to hold the initial 1 to 2 torr. When gas evolution is substantially completed, the current is slowly raised to about 1 A to decompose the metal carbonates. This process should be complete when the cathode shell reaches a dull red (about 1000°C) for a minute. When the CO_2 evolved from the carbonate decomposition is pumped, a final fill of tank oxygen is admitted to complete the oxide conversion. The current is again raised to a value which briefly brings the cathode shell to a dull red heat. Very little change in system pressure should occur during this step. It is important to avoid running large processing-discharge currents any longer than necessary, for two reasons: rapid evaporation of cathode coating occurs, and overheating and collapse of the seal-off constriction is likely. The latter can be monitored by clipping a piece of tissue paper around the constriction. When the tissue begins to turn brown, glass collapse is imminent. There is some evidence in favor of a final cathode processing using a glow discharge in pure hydrogen to form a monatomic layer of pure barium, but satisfactory performance has been obtained by omitting this step.

The tubes are then pumped for 36 hr at less than 10^{-6} torr with a hot blanket cover (approximately 150°C). Fill with spectroscopic-grade natural helium-neon (9:1) to a pressure of 1.5 to 2 torr, and process the anodes to the vacuum station cathode at 100 mA for 1 hr. Pump out hard and rf-discharge the reservoirs until glass-wall fluorescence is observed. Refill the tube with helium-neon and operate with normal discharge current, using the tube cathode for at least 24 hr—the longer the better. Pump hard again and flash the getter. Final gas filling of the helium 3–neon 20 isotopes is now made. The optimum pressure is approximately $4/d$ torr, where d is the tube diameter in millimeters. Check the operation with normal discharge conditions, and make the final seal-off.

Much of the processing procedure described in the section on glow-discharge plasma tubes is applicable to the arc tubes. The goal is the same, to remove as much of the impurity gas from the plasma tube and associated structures as possible. One of the effective ways of cleaning the surfaces is to use a low-pressure glow discharge in helium with the water-cooling jacket empty. A neon-sign transformer is ideally suited for this purpose, since it provides automatic current limiting and makes the normal anode and cathode surfaces alternate as cold cathodes for the glow discharge. By adjusting the helium pressure, the glow can be made to cover the entire plasma-tube surface, including the metal structures. This glow-discharge cleaning process is repeated by pumping and refilling with helium until the gas stays clean. Care should be taken to keep sputtering of the metal parts to a minimum to avoid window contamination. If the plasma tube employs a commercial oxide cathode, it may now be processed according to the manufacturer's instructions. If the experimental lanthanum hexaboride cathode is used, the heater is slowly raised to its operating temperature (about 1550°C) to outgas and sinter the coating. The cathode is then ready for operation. The water-cooling jacket is filled, and the first fill of reagent-grade gas is made. The first few fillings should be somewhat higher than normal operating pressures and be discarded as impurities appear. During this run-in period, the buildup of molecular impurity gases tends to cause discharge instabilities, and it is advisable initially to limit the current-to-threshold values with large ballast resistors. As the impurity evolution rate decreases with repeated pumping and filling, the arc currents are increased to their normal full-power levels, with the ballast resistor gradually being adjusted to its minimum value. The rates of impurity evolution and gas-fill cleanup are both asymptotic to a value depending on plasma-tube parameters. For sealed-off tubes, a knowledge of this value will determine the getter capacity required to keep the tube clean, as well as the storage or leak rate required to maintain the pressure. For experimental tubes remaining on the vacuum station, the extra complication of getters and leak valves is unnecessary.

The construction of pulsed-mercury plasma tubes was discussed in Section 7–1. The vacuum processing of the pulsed positive-column tube is perhaps the simplest of all gas lasers. In fact, adequate operation may be obtained with only a mechanical forepump and several torr of welding-grade helium. The cold oxide cathodes are processed first. Make sure that the mercury reservoir is cold-trapped at this time. The final cathode processing is done with 1 to 2 torr of helium, with repeated pumping and refilling until a clean helium discharge is observed. Close the stopcock, and allow the mercury to reach room temperature or slightly above. Laser action at 5677 Å will slowly build up as the mercury diffuses through the discharge. The windows may be kept clear of condensation by small tape heaters set at about 60 to 80°C. Ball joints allow easy adjustment of Brewster's angle and skew for optimum output. The gain is ample enough to use metal-coated mirrors for the optical resonator. The plasma tube shown is easily aligned with mirrors of 3-m radius of curvature.

The hollow-cathode plasma tube may be vacuum-processed with either natural mercury or the cheapest isotope, mercury 202. The procedures are nearly identical, except that special precautions are necessary to ensure that the valuable isotope is not pumped away during processing, and the plasma-tube structure is exceptionally clean to avoid gettering of impurities by the expensive isotope vapor. The processing configuration is shown in Figure 7-9, along with the optical cavity, so that laser operation may be obtained on the vacuum station. This technique provides the ultimate check on correct procedures, with the final tip-off being delayed until the laser displays stable operation.

The hollow-cathode plasma tube is assumed to have been fabricated and cleaned according to the recipe of Section 7–1. The glassing operation to the vacuum station is made through a drying tube after purging with dry nitrogen. The system is pumped down to forepump pressures and is leak-checked. If the system is leak-free, dry nitrogen is admitted to atmospheric pressure, and the mercury-filling reservoir cap is carefully blown open. Using a glass dropper, carefully insert a ball of instrument-grade mercury. About 100 mg (if the isotope is used, 25 mg) will suffice with careful processing. The reservoir

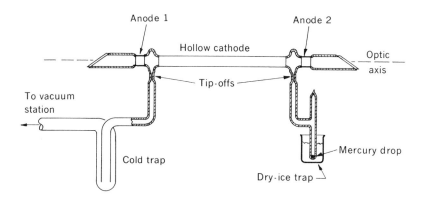

FIG. 7-9.   A mercury-ion-laser vacuum processing arrangement.

cap is then tipped off, and a small dry-ice trap is mounted to ensure no loss of mercury during the final processing. This is especially important to conserve the isotope, if used. The system is now pumped hard (10^{-6} torr or more) for several hours, leaving the cold trap on the mercury but not on the pumping tip-off side. Admit about 1 torr of reagent-grade helium, and connect the processing glow-discharge supply to anode 2($+$) of the mercury plasma tube and ($-$) to the cathode on the vacuum manifold. The helium plasma will effectively remove the adsorbed impurities from the walls. The buildup of these impurities can be monitored as band spectra superimposed on the helium sharp-line spectrum by using a pocket spectroscope looking along the axis of the plasma tube. The first discharge will usually become "dirty" within a few minutes and will require repumping and a fresh charge of clean helium. After several purges, the gas should stay clean for an indefinite period. At this point, a final leak check with acetone is made at the seals while monitoring with the hand spectroscope for hydrogen lines. The system is now ready for the final hard pumping, and the pumping tip-off cold trap is filled. The dry-ice mercury trap is removed, and the dry ice is transferred to the center of the hollow cathode. Avoid cooling of the glass to metal seals. The mercury will sublime from the reservoir and freeze out again in the cathode. Some gentle heat may be applied to ensure that all the mercury is sublimed. The mercury reservoir may now be tipped off and leak-checked. The pressure should remain in the 10^{-6}-torr region during this operation. Pure reagent-grade helium is now admitted to the vacuum manifold with a pressure of 6 to 8 torr. At this point, the hollow cathode is allowed to warm up, and the plasma-tube pulser is connected. Oscillation on the 6150-Å line should build up strongly within a few minutes, at which point the pulser is turned off to avoid mercury migration before tip-off. The plasma tube is now processed, and the final sealing operation is completed.

7–4 POWER SUPPLIES FOR GAS LASERS

The excitation of gas-laser plasmas has been accomplished with a wide variety of power sources: direct-current, radio-frequency, microwave, capacitor-discharge, and occasionally combinations of these methods. The long positive columns associated with gas-laser plasmas present a number of design problems that require careful engineering to achieve noise-free optical outputs, especially with cw devices. A convenient division of the required exciter properties can be made by separating the gas-laser plasmas into two groups: the glow-discharge systems (characterized by modest currents and high voltage drops) and the arc systems (large currents and relatively low voltage drops). The pulsed plasmas, although complicated in their behavior, can be driven with simple capacitor discharge.

Because the excitation parameters for experimental plasma tubes are subject to such wide variation, this section will treat only typical power supplies for the more commonly used gas lasers; these may be modified as required.

It is worth noting that the larger exciters are capable of delivering potentially lethal shocks; and where possible, the circuits are arranged to be fully floating with respect to ground. The experimenter should avoid working on concrete floors and should isolate the experimental plasma tube from spurious leakage paths, such as cooling water and gas discharges through the vacuum manifold. Permitting the latter to happen, especially with pulsed plasmas, is a common way of destroying some of the pressure-gauge circuits.

The helium-neon system requires power-supply design criteria which are typical for glow-discharge plasma tubes. The long, highly confined positive column is most easily driven by a ballasted direct-current source similar to that shown in Figure 7-10.

There is a tendency to generate plasma oscillations with long bores, and the circuit should keep stray capacitances at the electrodes to a minimum by closely connected ballast resistors. The superposition of radio-frequency electric fields along the outside of the bore wall is very effective in suppressing plasma noise and contributes a slight improvement in the output power of the helium-neon laser.

Radio-frequency excitation is also preferred when exciting mixtures of gases whose ionization potentials differ markedly, for example, helium and xenon. In this case direct-current excitation is unacceptable because of the separation of the gases by cataphoresis—the gas with lowest ionization potential (xenon) accumulating at the cathode.

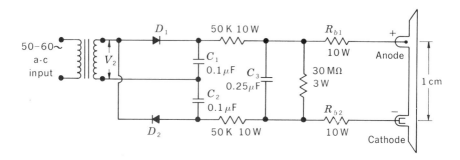

FIG. 7-10. A typical glow-discharge supply (V_2 rms $\approx$ 50 × 1 cm, volts; capacity rating, $C_1 + C_2 = C_3 = 4V_2$; ballast value, $R_{B1} + R_{B2} \approx$ 3K × 1 cm).

The effective negative resistance of a typical helium-neon plasma tube is shown in Figure 7-11. To achieve discharge stability, the positive impedance of the ballast must be equal to or greater than this value from 0 to about 100 kc. The effect of power-supply current ripple is comparatively small. Near saturation, the system exhibits very little modulation of the laser light output, even with a peak-to-peak ripple as high as 20 percent.

The argon-ion laser requires power-supply design criteria which are typical for arc discharges in the noble gases. When excited by direct current,

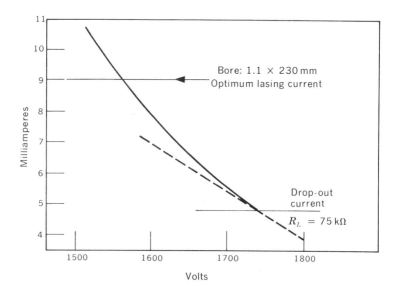

FIG. 7-11. Typical V-/ characteristics of a glow discharge.

these long positive columns do not show the usual negative resistance characteristic of the short arc lamps and, in principle, can be operated without a series stabilizing resistor. However, experience has shown that any slight change in plasma properties which may arise from pressure changes, impurities, magnetic-field fluctuations, and so on, causes a transient in the arc sustaining voltage which usually extinguishes the discharge unless some current stabilization is employed. The effect diminishes with increasing current density and increasing gas pressure.

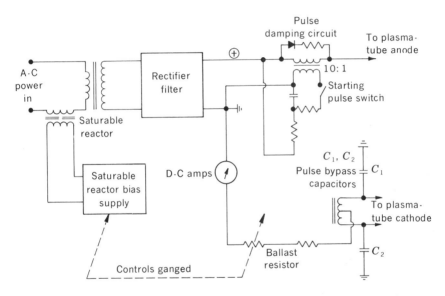

FIG. 7-12.   A typical direct-current supply for ion lasers.

Arc-discharge supplies are required to deliver substantial amounts of direct-current power, and should be well-engineered with interlocks and protective circuits to safeguard the plasma tube from being damaged. A power-supply design that provides excellent operating stability over the entire range of operating current is shown in the block diagram of Figure 7-12.

The system uses a saturable reactor as the input power control, ganged with a variable ballast resistor. The saturable reactor is attractive in two respects: it provides maximum open-circuit voltage for easy starting, yet is automatically current-limited under any short-circuit conditions. The initial starting pulse is provided by a capacitor discharge through a tertiary winding on the final filter choke. To ensure reliable striking, the pulse should last at least 0.1 msec and deliver a current of several amperes. It is important to damp out the ringing of the choke primary with a diode and resistor to ensure that the main power supply will take over the discharge when the starting pulse decays. A well-designed power supply should be interlocked in such a way as to provide maximum protection for the plasma tube. The suggested interlock sequence should be (1) cooling water flow, (2) cathode heater current, (3) magnet current, (4) maximum ballast resistance, (5) striking pulse, and finally (6) operating discharge current.

Arc discharges may also be excited at radio frequencies by induction coupling to the H field of a high-powered oscillator tank coil. Although the power supply is considerably more complex than the dc supply, the scheme has the advantage of eliminating all plasma-tube electrodes, permitting reactive vapors such as sulfur and chlorine to be excited. An effective way of coupling the radio-frequency energy to the long-arc column is a closed-loop gas ring discharge. The arrangement may be considered as an rf transformer, coupled to a one-turn secondary which constitutes the load. Because the gas-discharge load has both resistive and reactive components which change with the plasma-current density, the primary tank coil must be retuned to maintain optimum coupling as a function of power level. If one operates at fixed frequency with an oscillator-amplifier combination, the output tank circuit constants must be changed. Alternatively, the tank circuit constants can remain fixed, and the oscillator frequency be returned. The latter situation can be automatically achieved by making the tank circuit the frequency-determining element of a high-powered free-running class C oscillator. Experience with this form of exciter has shown that the coupling to the load is so effective that very little radiation occurs, despite the high levels of rf power generated. A typical circuit used with a ring-discharge plasma tube is shown in Figure 7-13. With the components shown, the oscillation frequency typically will be between 8 and 12 Mc and will drive an argon-ion laser to several watts output. Several points in the circuit design are worth noting. The positive ground keeps dangerous dc voltages away from the tank circuit and simplifies cooling of the triode anode and tank coil. Electrostatic shields are provided between the tank coil and the plasma tube to suppress E-field losses to the plasma and cooling jacket. The overall efficiency for dc power into power in the bore is about 50 percent.

Capacitive discharges combined with pulse-shaping networks and high-current switches provide a powerful technique for the study of the transient behavior of plasmas. In its simplest form, the plasma tube itself can serve as the switch, provided that the ratio of breakdown to sustaining voltage across the discharge is at least 2:1 and that sufficient time is allowed for deionization. These self-relaxing gas-discharge oscillators tend to be sporadic in their behavior, however, and more sophisticated pulse modulators are necessary

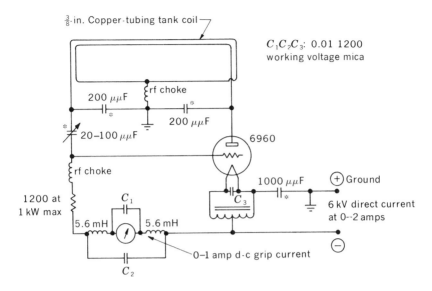

FIG. 7-13. A typical radio-frequency supply for gas-ion lasers.
(*: these capacitors are all 20-kV vacuum-ceramic.)

when careful control of pulse power and shape are desired. The most versatile
pulse modulator for experimental plasma tubes is the type commonly used to
drive radar magnetrons. These may contain either hydrogen thyratrons or
large high-vacuum tubes as switches and can provide pulse powers approaching 1 MW when properly matched. Because gas-discharge load impedances

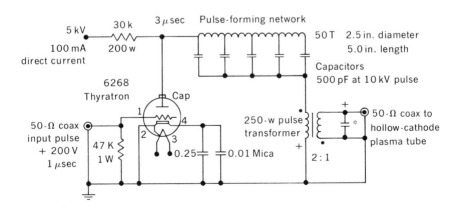

FIG. 7-14. A typical hollow-cathode pulsed supply for the mercury-ion
laser. (*: capacitor $\approx$ 0.05 μF, chosen to optimize rise time for a given
coax cable length.)

are subject to such wide variation, high-vacuum triode switches are preferred since they effectively decouple the plasma from the driver when the switch is off. Hydrogen thyratrons are simple and efficient and can be used when well-matched to a known load. Protective circuits should be provided to prevent spurious triggering in the event that some mismatch occurs. An example of a small thyratron pulse modulator for driving the hollow-cathode mercury-ion laser is shown in Figure 7-14. The driving-pulse parameters and the laser output are plotted in Figure 7-15.

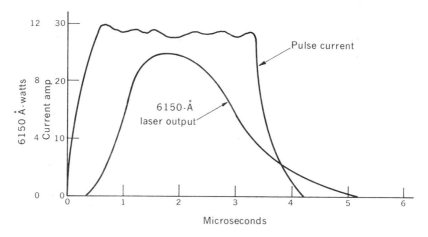

FIG. 7-15.   Mercury-ion-laser output pulse versus current.

7–5   MIRRORS AND WINDOWS FOR GAS LASERS

Apart from the plasma tube, the most critical components in a gas laser are the mirrors and windows comprising the optical cavity. Considerable progress has been made in the production of very high-quality optical components since the advent of the gas laser; in this section we shall review the current state of the art.

The subject of laser optical components can be subdivided into two areas: (1) the fabrication of the components from raw stock and (2) the coating of finished components for specific purposes.

The fabrication of laser mirrors and windows can be accomplished by using standard optical-shop practice. The tolerance on the figure of these components is moderately stringent: as a general rule, the deviations from a desired surface figure should be held to less than $\frac{1}{20}\lambda$ over the size of the laser beam incident on them. The most important specification on laser mirrors and windows, however, is with regard to the tolerable surface scatter. Surface scatter, since it introduces undesirable loss in laser cavities, should be held to an absolute minimum. Typically, this is accomplished by rather long (~24 hr) final polishing of the components.

Mirrors for use in gas lasers are usually coated with multilayer dielectric films. Of the various designs that have been used, the most common is the

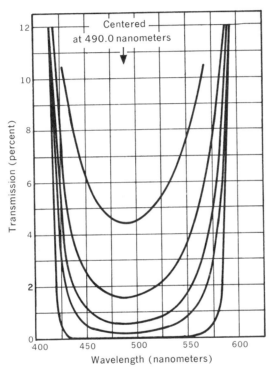

FIG. 7-16. Characteristics of high-reflectance laser mirrors. The different curves pertain to mirrors having different numbers of layers.

so-called "quarter-wave stack," which consists of alternate high- and low-index materials, each having an optical thickness of $\frac{1}{4}\lambda$. The transmission of such a coating is shown in Figure 7-16. The different curves in this figure pertain to coatings with different numbers of layers.

Absorption and scattering losses in good-quality quarter-wave stacks are typically on the order of 0.2 percent; and with care, these can be reduced to less than 0.1 percent. It is thus possible to obtain mirrors with reflectances on the order of 99.8 percent routinely, and undoubtedly reflectances of 99.9 percent will become common in the near future.

In addition to high-reflectance coatings, antireflection coatings are often used in gas-laser systems. The most common antireflection coating for laser use is the "V coat," which is a two-layer coating comprising a high- and a low-index film. The reflectance of a typical V coat is shown in Figure 7-17.

Coating technology is currently advancing at a rapid pace, and it is likely that in the near future the number of different types of coatings suitable for use in lasers will be increased considerably. For example, laser-quality

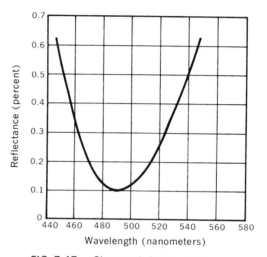

FIG. 7-17.   Characteristics of a "V" coat.

broadband high-reflectance coatings are currently undergoing extensive development, as are laser-quality broadband antireflection coatings.

Most high-quality laser mirrors in use today are so-called "hard" coatings, using materials such as TiO_2 and SiO_2. In the early days of laser research, mirror coatings were made using "soft" materials such as ZnS and cryolite, because these materials had low scatter loss. Coating technology has since progressed through several intermediate-hardness materials to the point where hard coatings are of equal quality to the older soft coatings. The advantage of hard coatings is, of course, that they are durable and can be readily cleaned.

7–6   MECHANICAL CONSTRUCTION OF GAS LASERS

The mechanical design of gas lasers represents a challenging problem in engineering. The mechanical structure of a laser must have the number of degrees of freedom necessary for the proper positioning of the mirrors and plasma tube, should be free from vibration, and should be thermally stable. In an ideal situation, both the separation and angular orientation of the laser mirrors would remain constant as the structure heats up (primarily, because of heat generated by the gas discharge). In practice, it is extremely difficult to design a laser which meets both these criteria. Angularly stable structures are not too difficult to design, but structures of appropriate size for gas lasers, which maintain length stability to a small fraction of an optical wavelength as the ambient temperature changes by several degrees, are very difficult to design.

The degree of sophistication required in the mechanical design of a gas laser depends on the intended use of the laser. Thus, lasers which are intended to maintain alignment for several months, or years, require more attention to mechanical design than do laboratory lasers, which can be aligned daily.

In general, the mechanical design of lasers should follow kinematic principles, so that adjustable parts are not overconstrained. One of the major problems that appears in typical gas lasers is warpage of the structure resulting from thermal gradients. Often this problem can be reduced by kinematic mounting of the various parts. In extreme cases, it may be desirable to place a heat shield between the laser structure and the plasma tube in order to cut down thermal gradients.

It is generally necessary to set the angular orientation of the mirrors to within several seconds of arc. Many elaborate mirror mounts have been invented to do this, but with a modicum of effort, it is possible to design satisfactory simple mounts using conventional screws and spring-loaded washers.

Two materials, aluminum and Invar, are commonly used for gas-laser structures. Invar has the advantage of low thermal expansion but has a low thermal conductivity. Aluminum, on the other hand, has a large thermal-expansion coefficient, but it also has a high thermal conductivity, so that it is more difficult to set up thermal gradients in aluminum than it is in Invar. As far as angularly stable structures are concerned, the two materials are more or less equivalent. For lasers designed to have length stability, Invar is the better material; unfortunately, it is more difficult to obtain and is considerably more expensive.

REFERENCES

A fully adequate list of references for this chapter would include hundreds of listings. We give only two that have been found particularly useful.

1. W. H. Kohl, "Handbook of Materials and Techniques for Vacuum Devices," Reinhold Publishing Corporation, New York, 1967.

This is a good general reference book for plasma-tube construction. It contains a great deal of information not available anywhere else.

2. S. Dushman, "Scientific Foundations of Vacuum Technique," 2d ed., John Wiley & Sons, Inc., New York, 1962.

This is the standard reference on vacuum technique.

Some Formulas from Electromagnetic Theory

The basic equations of electromagnetic theory are Maxwell's equations:

$$\operatorname{div} \vec{D} = \rho \tag{A1-1}$$

$$\operatorname{div} \vec{B} = 0 \tag{A1-2}$$

$$\operatorname{curl} \vec{E} = -\frac{\partial \vec{B}}{\partial t} \tag{A1-3}$$

$$\operatorname{curl} \vec{H} = \vec{J} + \frac{\partial \vec{D}}{\partial t} \tag{A1-4}$$

The vectors $\vec{D}$, $\vec{B}$, $\vec{E}$, and $\vec{H}$ appearing in these equations are called the "electric displacement," the "magnetic induction," the "electric intensity," and the "magnetic intensity," respectively. $\vec{J}$ is the current density, and ρ is the charge density.

The vectors $\vec{D}$ and $\vec{H}$ are related to $\vec{E}$ and $\vec{B}$ by

$$\vec{D} = \epsilon_0 \vec{E} + \vec{P} \tag{A1-5}$$

$$\vec{H} = \frac{1}{\mu_0} \vec{B} - \vec{M} \tag{A1-6}$$

The constants ϵ_0 and μ_0 appearing in these equations are called the "permittivity of free space" and the "permeability of free space." They have the following numerical values:

$$\epsilon_0 = 8.85 \times 10^{-12} \quad \text{farad/meter} \tag{A1-7}$$

$$\mu_0 = 4\pi \times 10^{-7} \quad \text{henry/meter} \tag{A1-8}$$

The vectors $\vec{P}$ and $\vec{M}$ in Eqs. (A1-5) and (A1-6) are called the "electric polarization" and the "magnetic polarization." In the optical region of the spectrum, the magnitude of the magnetic polarization is negligible.

In an isotropic material, the vectors $\vec{D}$ and $\vec{H}$ are parallel to $\vec{E}$ and $\vec{B}$, respectively, so that we have

$$\vec{D} = \epsilon\vec{E} \tag{A1-9}$$

$$\vec{H} = \frac{1}{\mu}\vec{B} \tag{A1-10}$$

The quantities ϵ and μ are called the "permittivity" and the "permeability" of the material.

The dielectric constant of a material is defined as

$$\kappa_e = \frac{\epsilon}{\epsilon_0} \tag{A1-11}$$

The polarization of a material is related to the electric intensity by the relation

$$\vec{P} = \chi\epsilon_0\vec{E} \tag{A1-12}$$

where χ is called the "electric susceptibility" of the material. In an isotropic material, χ is a scalar quantity. The susceptibility of a material is related to the dielectric constant by

$$\chi = \kappa_e - 1 \tag{A1-13}$$

In a conducting material, the current density is related to the electric intensity by

$$\vec{J} = \sigma\vec{E} \tag{A1-14}$$

where σ is the conductivity of the material.

In a homogeneous, isotropic material containing no net charge density, the electric intensity must obey a wave equation

$$\nabla^2\vec{E} - \mu_0\sigma\frac{\partial\vec{E}}{\partial t} - \epsilon_0\mu_0\frac{\partial^2\vec{E}}{\partial t^2} = \mu_0\frac{\partial^2\vec{P}}{\partial t^2} \tag{A1-15}$$

In order to study the general solution of Eq. (A1-15), it is convenient to eliminate the explicit appearance of the polarization. Using Eqs. (A1-11), (A1-12), and (A1-13), we find that

$$\nabla^2 \vec{E} - \mu_0 \sigma \frac{\partial \vec{E}}{\partial t} - \kappa_e \epsilon_0 \mu_0 \frac{\partial^2 \vec{E}}{\partial t^2} = 0 \qquad \text{(A1-16)}$$

In order to further simplify the study of the solution, we assume that we can represent the electric intensity by a scalar quantity E. This scalar quantity can be interpreted as a single component of the vector electric intensity. A plane-wave solution of Eq. (A1-16) is

$$E(z, t) = E_0 e^{i(k_c z - \omega t)} \qquad \text{(A1-17)}$$

where E_0 and k_c are complex quantities. E_0 is called the "complex amplitude," k_c is called the "complex wave number," and ω is called the "angular frequency" of the wave. The actual electric intensity E is given by the real part of the above expression. In order for Eq. (A1-17) to be a solution of (A1-16), the complex wave number must satisfy the equation

$$k_c{}^2 = \frac{\omega^2}{c^2} \left(\kappa_e + i \frac{\sigma}{\epsilon_0 \omega} \right) \qquad \text{(A1-18)}$$

where we have made explicit note in this equation that in free space the wave propagates with a velocity

$$c = \frac{1}{\sqrt{\epsilon_0 \mu_0}} \qquad \text{(A1-19)}$$

We are led from Eq. (A1-18) to define a complex dielectric constant

$$\kappa_{ec} \equiv \kappa_e + i \frac{\sigma}{\epsilon_0 \omega} \qquad \text{(A1-20)}$$

The complex refractive index of a material is then defined by

$$n_c{}^2 \equiv \kappa_{ec} = \kappa_e + i \frac{\sigma}{\epsilon_0 \omega} \qquad \text{(A1-21)}$$

The complex refractive index is written in terms of its real and imaginary parts as

$$n_c = n + i\kappa \qquad \text{(A1-22)}$$

In this expression, n is called the "refractive index," and κ is called the "attenuation index." Note that the attenuation index κ is not to be confused with the dielectric constant κ_e.

By analogy with Eq. (A1-13), one is also led to define a complex susceptibility

$$\chi_c = \kappa_{ec} - 1 \qquad \text{(A1-23)}$$

where χ_c is conventionally written in terms of its real and imaginary parts as

$$\chi_c = \chi' + i\chi'' \qquad \text{(A1-24)}$$

Noting from Eqs. (A1-18) and (A1-21) that

$$k_c = \frac{\omega}{c} n_c \qquad \text{(A1-25)}$$

we write

$$E = E_0 e^{-(\omega/c)\kappa z} e^{i[(\omega/c)nz - \omega t]} \qquad \text{(A1-26)}$$

The solution of Eq. (A1-16) is now seen to be an exponentially damped wave. The wave number of the wave is

$$k = \frac{\omega}{c} n \qquad \text{(A1-27)}$$

and the wavelength is

$$\lambda \equiv 2\pi k \qquad \text{(A1-28)}$$

The absorption coefficient of the material is defined as

$$\alpha \equiv \frac{2\omega}{c} \kappa \qquad \text{(A1-29)}$$

It is often convenient to express the absorption coefficient in terms of the susceptibility of the material. Using Eqs. (A1-22), (A1-23), and (A1-24), we see that

$$\alpha = \frac{\omega}{c} \chi'' \qquad \text{(A1-30)}$$

The gain per unit length g_l (the gain coefficient) is the negative of the absorption coefficient. Thus,

$$g_l = -\alpha = -\frac{\omega}{c} \chi'' \qquad \text{(A1-31)}$$

The refractive index for a *weakly* absorbing material can be written in terms of the susceptibility by noting that

$$\kappa_{ec} = n_c^2 \approx n^2 + i2\kappa \qquad \text{(A1-32)}$$

so that

$$n \approx 1 + \tfrac{1}{2}\chi' \qquad \text{(A1-33)}$$

The flow of energy in an electromagnetic field is described by using the Poynting vector, which is defined as

$$\vec{S} \equiv \vec{E} \times \vec{H} \qquad \text{(A1-34)}$$

In free space the magnitude of the electric intensity is related to the magnitude of the magnetic intensity by

$$H = \sqrt{\frac{\epsilon_0}{\mu_0}}\, E \qquad\qquad \text{(A1-35)}$$

The power/area in an electromagnetic wave is the time average of the Poynting vector. In free space this is given by

$$W = \frac{c\epsilon_0}{2}\, E^*E \qquad\qquad \text{(A1-36)}$$

As was shown in Chapter 2, the gain coefficient and refractive index of a radiative transition in a gas can be expressed in terms of a function called the "plasma dispersion function." In this appendix, we shall summarize some useful properties of the plasma dispersion function. For a more extensive discussion, including a table of the plasma dispersion function, the reader is referred to the book by Fried and Conte.[1]

The plasma dispersion function may be defined by

$$Z(\zeta) = \frac{2\zeta}{\sqrt{\pi}} \int_0^\infty \frac{e^{-t^2}}{t^2 - \zeta^2} \, dt \qquad (A2\text{-}1)$$

where

$$\zeta = \xi + i\eta \qquad \eta > 0 \qquad (A2\text{-}2)$$

It is related to the error function of a complex argument $W(\zeta)$ by[2]

$$Z(\zeta) = i\sqrt{\pi} \, W(\zeta) \qquad (A2\text{-}3)$$

The function has the following power-series expansion:

$$Z(\zeta) \approx i\sqrt{\pi} \, e^{-\zeta^2} - 2\zeta + \tfrac{4}{3}\zeta^3 - \tfrac{8}{15}\zeta^5 + \cdots \qquad (A2\text{-}4)$$

[1] B. D. Fried and S. D. Conte, "The Plasma Dispersion Function" (The Hilbert Transform of the Gaussian), Academic Press, Inc., New York, 1961.

[2] The error function of a complex argument is tabulated in Abramowitz and Stegun, "Handbook of Mathematical Functions," Dover Publications, New York, 1965.

and the following asymptotic expansion for $\eta > 0$:

$$Z(\zeta) \approx -\frac{1}{\zeta}\left[1 + \frac{1}{2\zeta^2} + \frac{3}{4\zeta^4} + \cdots\right] \tag{A2-5}$$

For $\eta = 0$, the function becomes

$$Z(\xi) = i\sqrt{\pi}\,e^{-\xi^2} - 2e^{-\xi^2}\int_0^\xi e^{t^2}\,dt \tag{A2-6}$$

INDEX